CW00853965

Spire Publishing
www.spirepublishing.com

The Daily Trials Of Living With Fibromyalgia
&
Arthritic Pain

by
Angela J Coupar

Spire Publishing
www.spirepublishing.com

First published in Canada 2007 by Angela J Coupar.

The moral right of Angela J Coupar to be identified as the author of this work has been asserted.

Designed in Toronto, Canada by Adlibbed ltd.
Publishing services supplied by spirepublishing.com
Printed and bound by Lightningsource in the US or the UK.

ISBN: 1-897312-42-3

Disclaimer

This book has been written from my own experience of having the condition Fibromyalgia and more recently Osteoarthritis. I the author hereby write notice that I am not medically qualified. The information presented in this book contains material I have read and researched myself and is for informational purposes only. I make no claim to the information being able to reduce or eradicate the condition Fibromyalgia, Osteoarthritis, or any other condition mentioned within these contents. Neither, do I take any responsibility for the information mentioned within this book used as reference from other persons and/or companies.

The information and suggestions within this book should not be replaced by the services or medication prescribed by your medical doctor or, should it be administered without their knowledge and advice. All matters regarding health require medical supervision, and any application of treatments, alternative or conventional set forth within this book are at the reader's own risk. I the author cannot be held responsible.

"To everyone who has ever given me inspiration to continue this journey of life"

Dedication:

Dad, you never recovered enough to be able to read the final manuscript, but I know you would be proud of the finished book, and of my achievements.

In Loving Memory of

John Mander – Aged 68
1938 – 2006

Loved, Cherished & Always In Our Hearts

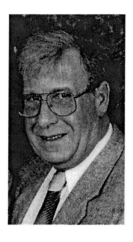

Your love, understanding words and memories of your warm smile bring so much comfort

Forever Missed & Never Forgotten

XXX

Authors Note:

Having Fibromyalgia doesn't mean life should come to a stop, although with this condition living a normal existence may seem daunting, especially where employment and everyday issues are concerned. However, I do know and understand how hard it can be with the discomfort and pain this condition creates, although compared to some sufferers I am thankful that I do not have it in its most severe form which can warrant the use of crutches or a wheel chair. At the time of writing this publication I coped with many bad days, but also some positive days where I felt almost normal and ailment free... However, on the whole my FMS continues to be a daily annoyance of discomfort and pain, although bearable to a point, most of the time.

Like everyone else with Fibromyalgia, some days are worse than others and at times it seems that there are more bad days than good with that pill bottle and other treatments working overtime. However, please take a leaf from my book and keep smiling and laughing. Happiness is one of the greatest healers... So keep on looking for that 'Spark of Light' through the fog and your days will feel much better...

During the writing of this book, I was also diagnosed with Osteoarthritis and although this book mainly covers the condition fibromyalgia, you will find many tips on alternative therapies that may help various forms of arthritis throughout this publication.

Making the most out of your life will help too see you through the not so good days.
Life is one big journey and no matter how you suffer, there is always someone much worse off than your self...

I hope that you find the information in my book not only interesting, but helpful.

Content

Authors Note   Page 10

Acknowledgements   Page 13

About The Author   Page 14

Introduction   Page 15

Understanding Fibromyalgia   Page 21

How I Manage My FMS   Page 27

What exactly is Fibromyalgia   Page 42

How to Diagnose Fibromyalgia   Page 50

Fibromyalgia Symptoms   Page 54

Alternative Remedies   Page 58

Crystal Healing   Page 78

Conventional Treatments   Page 83

Fibromyalgia and Sex   Page 88

My Fibro A-Z   Page 93

A Letter to the Normals   Page 105

Fibro Messages   Page 108

Authors Final Word   Page 116

Key Words   Page 121

References   Page 123

Recommended FMS Related Publications   Page 126

Recommended Arthrtis Related Publications Page 128

Fibromyalgia & Arthritis Resources   Page 130

Authors Other Book   Page 135

<u>Acknowledgements</u>

To my loving husband, who is continually by my side and understanding through the good and bad days, and to our beautiful Border Collies, Elsie & Wilma, Galahad the Welsh Mountain pony and Casper the Shetland pony who bring endless amounts of happiness to us everyday. Also to my dad, mum, brother and parent-in-laws for their continued support and understanding over the years, I love and appreciate you all.

To everyone, who has ever suffered with Fibromyalgia, any other form of Arthritis or Rheumatism, Chronic Fatigue Syndrome, or one of the numerous conditions that have similar symptoms – your experiences will bring understanding to others in the future and to those that research these conditions in the hope of finding a treatment that will alleviate the suffering of those people now and in the future who are affected by these conditions.

To those people of whom I have never met, but through their own individual talents of either acting or producing music that either, make me laugh or sing, I thank you for making a difference. Happiness and Inspiration is such a healer in our journey of life…

And finally, with many thanks to everyone who took the time to proof read my manuscript, a daunting task for even the most patient.

"Of all the gifts that a wise providence grants us to make life full and happy, friendship is the most beautiful."

About The Author

Angela J Coupar lives with her husband, Border Collies, pet hamsters, a Welsh 'Section A' Mountain pony and Shetland pony, as well as the various animals that visit through Acre Fen Canine Crèche, and the hamsters who take refuge at Hamster Rescue (UK). Her love and devotion to caring for any animal is plain to see and all that pass through her door enjoy their experience.

Angela manages to place her fibromyalgia and osteoarthritis in the back seat as much as possible, and focuses her energy on making sure that all her animal guests are happy, have fun and have that all important understanding and love. In many respects, combined with her interests in alternative treatments and the few conventional medications she takes, I believe this is what keeps her motivated and determined not to let these conditions get in the way of the things she wants to do. Even when she is tired and enduring a day of painful discomfort, Angela still has a radiant smile that just glows with positive energy.

Angela has a certificate in Dog Pyschology and works from home, which enables her to manage her fibromyalgia and osteoarthritis more effectively. She has written one other book "Canine Behaviour Practice: A short guide to setting up your own business as a dog psychologist, behaviourist or therapist" and now works part time running her internet advice lines. She gives inspiration to others to manage their conditions and is determined to provide some help and advice through this book, using her own experiences.

G.C.

Introduction:

Hi… I'm Angela, a Fibromyalgia (FMS) sufferer for the past several years and more recently in September 2006 when I received the diagnosis that I also had Osteoarthritis*.

I decided to explain my condition in this book from when my fibromyalgia symptoms became more noticeable and medical support was introduced. However, I personally believe that I may have suffered with this condition well before 1999 as painful joints, muscles and ligaments were present for many years prior to this date.

Having a personal account of these conditions, I decided to put my experiences to paper and write this book. I am sure that you do not want an entire account of my life as this book would end up more like a volume of encyclopaedias which is not the point I want to make, but simply just to highlight the main target areas of how I manage my symptoms, with the hope that it will inspire others into helping themselves cope with the painful syndrome of FMS, and by also adding some information points on this particular condition. Browsing many book stores, it appeared that there were plenty of books written by the medical profession or those that simply research this condition, but very few books are available from those that experience the daily battle of coping with FMS. So here is my experience and tips for coping with the daily life of living with fibromyalgia and other arthritic conditions. I hope you enjoy the read.

Personally, I am a big fan of treating any personal or health condition holistically, whether the problem is depression, a common cold or my own fibromyalgia and osteoarthritis. Throughout this book I will explain the alternative treatments I have used and still do, as I believe they along with some more conventional medications have helped me to cope with this condition, although none of them singularly or combined are a cure – not for me anyway. Naturally, the treatments I use will not suit everyone and as with most treatments, they don't work for everyone. However, my philosophy is:

"If you don't try, you won't know."

I am not sure what triggered the fibromyalgia, but it may have been the result of physical trauma. Over the years, I have been involved in an accident where the car that I was a passenger in skidded on some mud and rolled over into an embankment. I was only shocked and bruised, but it may have played an unknown part in the development of my fibromyalgia long before the symptoms made an appearance for the first time. During my various employments I have had jobs where heavy lifting was a constant back ache to say the least and finally during a job as a confectioner for a supermarket I had a nasty fall in one of the big freezers, landing on my back which resulted in me being on pain killers and off work for several weeks.

There seems a mixed response by those that research fibromyalgia too whether this condition is hereditary or not. Well who am I to say if this is the case, but one thing I do know is that family members on both my parent's side have suffered with various forms of arthritic conditions, ranging from rheumatism, rheumatoid arthritis, osteoarthritis to degenerative arthritis in various joints ranging from the toes, knees, hips to fingers and wrists. When put together, we are quite a medical case, or as some people would say a family of medical disasters, but because of the number of people in my family who do suffer with arthritic type conditions it certainly makes you wonder if there is a hereditary link. It certainly doesn't just affect those over the age of 40.

Spondylosis also occurs in our family. I myself was diagnosed with Spondylosis in the Summer of 1999 and for weeks, endured physiotherapy and acupuncture to try and relieve the symptoms in my spine and neck. This condition is degenerative and affects the lower cervical intervertebral discs and tends to be more common in middle-aged people. This condition occurs when one or more of the discs prolapse which can create these symptoms:

Pain in the neck and back region

Normal movement which can be limited

Pain that tends to be worse on waking

In severe cases, Cervical Spondylosis can on occasions also create symptoms such as numbness, pain and weakness in the person's arms.

It was around this time that the problems really started, with severe pain to the extent that I simply didn't want to move or do anything. I could have literally cried with the pain and discomfort. What I cannot remember is whether I suffered any trauma at this particular time, or if the condition just appeared at a similar time to the Spondylosis. At the time I fostered many dogs for a local charity, which meant that many had never learnt to walk to heel, so pulled and yanked at their leads, which would place a considerable strain on my own joints and soft tissues. However, as with most people, I just put my symptoms down to general wear and tear of the human body.

During this time I found it extremely difficult to settle at night, or when I did I would wake up feeling un-refreshed, and because of the discomfort I began suffering from disturbed sleep patterns. This meant being either extremely restless or not sleeping at all. My hips and neck would generate a pain that can not be easily explained, but can be best described as a sharp burning dagger like feeling, and my other limbs including, my fingers, wrists, elbows and knees would be irritatingly painful. When not painful, they would have a constant and uncomfortable sore, throbbing ache that remains with me to this present day. Feeling dizzy and even fainting from the pain and tiredness occurred on several occasions and still does when my energy levels get too low. These days I tend to be one step ahead and as soon as I start to feel light headed, dizzy or have blurred vision I will go and lie down. If I don't, I know I will end up in a heap on the floor where I pass out.

Having consulted my doctor, she made the decision to send me for further tests. Blood test after blood test kept resulting in a mixture of normal and abnormal readings that the doctors simply couldn't identify. Now this is unusual in the fact that routine laboratory tests usually reveal no abnormalities with FMS sufferers, although there has been some research where several clinical studies have revealed damage and irregularities in the shape of the red blood cells in people suffering with chronic fatigue syndrome and fibromyalgia. Apparently, this causes blockages in the blood flow through the capillaries, which results in insufficient oxygen getting to the sufferer's muscles and tissues, which is the cause of the pain and fatigue. I believe that one researcher is attempting to get his blood test approved internationally. If this happens, it could become a much-needed diagnostic test. With my self, depending on how I was suffering at the time of the blood tests seemed to have an effect on the percentage in the results from normal, slightly above normal readings to abnormal readings on the days that I had been in pain when having the blood samples taken. Well, I don't mind blood tests, but this can be a work of art for the poor nurse involved as my veins can at times seem to run on thin air, and getting a sample can be like getting blood out of a stone. It's a good job I don't feel faint at the sight of a needle. The resulting bruises made me look like a junkie at times and seemed to take forever to disappear.

So after several weeks of testing and the doctors finding no evidence of arthritis in any form or the detection of any viruses, etc, it was decided that I should be referred to a Rheumatology consultant. A long wait of several months and luckily only one cancelled appointment, I finally got to see the consultant who I must say was very thorough and understanding in his approach. Well you guessed it. I had more blood tests and was poked, prodded and pulled about yet again, which resulted in a diagnosis of general degenerative wear and tear. Medication was prescribed with further periods of physiotherapy and acupuncture, which I must admit did help in the short term, but as soon as it ceased the symptoms returned with more severity.

A few months after this appointment, my husband and I moved to West Sussex in the South of England. I tried to push the symptoms aside as no one likes to make an appointment with a new doctor as soon as they move into a new area. However, it got to the stage where I needed a new prescription of pain killers as the Ibrufen wasn't having any effect and I felt I needed some further advice. So again I endured the usual routine of having examinations and blood samples. The bloods replicated those previously taken. So again, I was sent to a new set of Rheumatology consultants who after several appointments and further tests where the tender points in my knees, hips, elbows, neck, etc, were examined, I was diagnosed as having FMS related symptoms, but at least they had now confirmed that I hadn't got Rheumatoid Arthritis*, ME or any other condition that resulted in similar symptoms to those I was experiencing. So there was some progress at last.

The consultant explained the condition and prescribed me some anti-depressant tablets (Amitriptyline), which can have a side effect of making you drowsy and tired. These were prescribed to try and regulate my sleep patterns. However, they had no effect and the irregular sleep patterns continued. Ironically, some of the other side effects of this medication are similar to those conditions that fibromyalgia sufferers can have, including dizziness, headaches, weakness and bowel complaints to name a few. I was also prescribed a different anti-inflammatory tablet (Co-codamol) to help with the pain and discomfort which helped initially, but these days rarely has the desired effect on the days when the pain and discomfort is severe, or as I like to refer it to as 'being above my normal average'.

It was arranged, that I was to be sent an appointment to see the consultant again to discuss my progress and was supplied some literature to read and follow, which at the time was helpful, but knowing what I do now with regards to this condition the information I was initially supplied could have, and more to the point should have been more informative. The appointment was made for several weeks later. I was seen by a different consultant who then referred me to a clinic dealing with fibromyalgia and other similar conditions. My consultant also requested that I should have an EMG Test/Nerve Conduction Study, but instead of an appointment, I received a letter in the Autumn of 2001 stating that there was a long waiting list of approximately 10-12 months. So basically, I never did get to the clinic as my circumstances changed again, and apart from this I had begun to feel rather despondent waiting for an appointment and felt like I was continually being passed from pillar to post instead of receiving the support I needed at that particular time. Researching fibromyalgia on the internet became my new source of information and help, and I must say I have learned such a lot from these cyber space resources and have made many new acquaintances with the same condition, and these individuals have helped me not to feel so isolated.

So for those of you who have read my book this far and are still unfamiliar with what FMS stands for, it is medically known as Fibromyalgia Syndrome and is the term used for a 'Rheumatic Type Condition', previously referred to as either 'Soft Tissue Rheumatism', 'Fibrosis', or 'Non-Articular Rheumatism'. Unlike the common form of 'Degenerative Arthritis', which involves the body's joints, fibromyalgia attacks the 'Soft Tissues' of the human body, such as the muscles, tendons and ligaments causing widespread musculoskeletal pain. This can be combined with several other health conditions which can make the FMS a real nightmare to cope with. This is something I will explain in more detail later on in this book.

*** Chapter Footnote:** More recently in May 2006 I was referred to a new Rheumatology consultant at the Grantham & District Hospital. Dr. V. V. Kaushik sent me for a bone scan, as more recent symptoms have indicated that there may also be another condition present, such as osteoarthritis or rheumatoid arthritis.*

"Achieving can only begin with Believing"

Understanding Fibromyalgia

I am now in my mid thirties, but more often than not on the bad days I feel years older, with severe aches and pains that move from one area to another. I think of it as a bit like a free spirit moving from one place to another as the discomfort moves unpredictably around your body. Others may say there is a gremlin on the move, but no matter how you try and describe this symptom the problem remains the same. For example, it can move from your hips one day to your neck the next. Rarely does the fibromyalgia affect just one area, but triggers discomfort and pain in various points around your body including, the fingers, wrists, toes and knees. To those that do not understand this condition, explaining that the discomfort travels brings disbelief, but those that do have this condition will only know too well that this is a realistic account. I think if the discomfort was permanently in one place, it would be so much easier to deal with, but when it travels from one area to another, then personally I believe the treatment becomes less effective.

Simple every day tasks such as, using an aerosol spray (e.g.: deodorant or hairspray), opening cans, using a pair of scissors, lifting a plate or mug, folding washing, doing up buttons, or zips on clothes, to turning the page of a book can create severe pain and discomfort. The little things most people use and take for granted, but think nothing of them can be unbearable to those with this condition.

With this, FMS sufferers and those closest to them will also be able to relate to some of the natural human side effects which accompany the fibromyalgia. This can range from intimate problems with loved ones to mood swings. The intimate problems will be discussed further in this book. However, one of the problems, notably the mood swings means that we can be extremely bad tempered and snap at the slightest annoyance, very emotional and irritable when the pain is bad, and frustrated from the excessive fatigue caused from the lack of delta sleep, night after night.

Delta sleep is the normal phase of sleep where your body naturally relaxes, repairs and re-energizes and something that FMS sufferers are deprived of. As for myself, on good nights I manage 4-5 hours of disturbed sleep and never wake up refreshed and often feeling like I've done a round in the boxing ring followed by an all night party in a night club. On the bad nights I am lucky to get 2-3 hours of restless sleep where I often wake every couple of hours in pain, so you can appreciate that over time patience runs thin and frustration from the lack of sleep naturally set in to your daily pattern, although I must say that I naturally cope with this probably better than some with this condition as I just happen to be one of those people that can get along on very little sleep. These days I class four hours as a good night of sleep and it's been a long time since I had a full 8 hours of blissful rest. So understandably, is it any wonder people with this condition don't feel like snuggling up to their loved one for a romantic evening, or simply joining in a not so funny joke! Ask yourself this question…

"Could you manage with very little sleep as well as being in constant pain and discomfort with out displaying some personality changes?"

I think if you are honest with yourself, the answer would simply be:

"No"

People often say they dream at night, well if I do I can't remember, but it is probably more to the fact that I don't go into a deep enough sleep to dream. Inevitably, those closest to you tend to be on the receiving end of your tiredness and exhaustion, so their understanding and patience is vitally important in helping any FMS sufferer through the worst periods of this condition. My own husband is very understanding, but at times even he is pushed to the limits with my moods. When I'm in a moody frame of mind, I'm best left alone to calm down, relax and channel the negative energies away and replace them with some positive energy. Family and friends should avoid constant and irritating comments such as:

"I see you're in a bad mood again"
or
"Miserable as usual. Don't tell me another bad day!"

Such negative remarks really do not help, and this is where some understanding is required from those closest to you.

Having family and friends who show very little or no support at all, or show no understanding will inevitably lead to problems in relationships and the person with this condition will feel even more isolated and less able to cope with their symptoms. If you feel that you and your condition are not understood by those closest to you then perhaps write them a letter to express your feelings and to help educate them. I have added a letter which is 'Copyright of www.fibrohugs.com - Written by Ronald J. Waller' further on in this book, which you are welcome to copy or get inspiration from to write your own version, but if you do use the letter in this book, please do use the copyright details in full as described in the footnote on the letter page. Alternatively, let them read this book and where possible, sit down and discuss how you feel.

Do I look any different?

Well no… On the outside, apart from looking tired, stiff, pale or washed out most of the time, I can look as normal as the next person, but more often than not on the inside I feel like hell has just been re-invented and yes, on occasions I do get frustrated and angry at the way I feel. Along with the discomfort, stiffness and pain of the FMS, I can be extremely clumsy at times, have a terrible memory and unless I write something down, you can guarantee I'll forget. I can find it hard to concentrate at times and I am nearly always cold, which is due to me being sensitive to the weather conditions. I am always glad when our cold, damp English Winters are replaced by some warm Spring sun and often dream of moving to a warmer climate in the future. The South of France being my top destination to live, but Italy and parts of America also appeal to me.

Like many people with fibromyalgia I used to ask myself that all important question.

"Why Me?"

Then when I sat down and thought about it, I would find my answer.

"Well Why Not!"

'Life is life', and you have to learn to accept what your life throws at you, whether it is good or bad. I am a strong believer that we make our own luck and destiny, it doesn't come naturally. So basically you can either mope about feeling sorry for yourself as I have done in the past, or you can make use of a situation and help others with your own understanding and experience on how they feel as I hope to do with this book and also with my fibromyalgia related website, which can be found at: *www.fibromyalgiaandarthritis.co.uk*

Knowing that there are others around the world that can relate to how you feel with this condition can help and in many cases can also stop you feeling so isolated at the times when you feel at your most negative.

"This is a genuine health condition, which affects thousands of people throughout the UK and millions of people worldwide."

Experiencing extremely low points can trigger depression which if not controlled can turn into one revolving vicious circle of negative experiences and fibro symptoms. However, when you do sit down in a more positive frame of mind and think about other people around you, there are always those who are much worse off than yourself. There are far too many people around the world who suffer with the most horrific health conditions, but still learn to cope with them. My heart goes out to these people, and I sincerely hope that they receive all the support that they require to help them through their own discomforts.

As for those of us that suffer with fibromyalgia, there is nothing worse than being told *"it's all in the mind"* or *"pull yourself together"* and *"Stop being such a Hypochondriac"*, by people who do not understand the physical and mental pain you are suffering, despite the fact that you can be at times curled up on the floor in agony. To most people if you look fine on the outside, they tend to believe you are healthy on the inside, but with FMS this is not the case.

"Fibromyalgia is often badly understood, with many sufferers often experiencing themselves being classed as 'neurotic' or as a 'hypochondriac'."

Unfortunately, there is still a small number in the medical profession who despite all the numerous blood tests, x-rays, pulling and prodding still do not understand or accept that this medical problem can create such pain without being picked up by the usual conventional techniques that they use on other symptoms. However, saying this, thankfully these unhelpful and negative experiences are finally becoming less frequent as the medical profession have really started taking note of the many thousands over the world that suffer from the symptoms caused by this very real condition. Then there is our own continued personal battle of anger and frustration of having to wait so long for medical appointments to arrive, only to have them cancelled and re-issued at a later date, but again these problems are being dealt with by the health service and government and I must confess that since I have been living in Lincolnshire and resuming my conventional medicine and treatments in 2006, hospital response times have greatly improved. The medical professionals who work at the Grantham & District hospital are not only very helpful, but appointments are issued promptly.

"FMS sufferers often 'outwardly' appear healthy, despite being in tremendous pain and discomfort."

However, from the time I decided to cancel out most conventional style medical help in the latter part of the year 2001 (*up until recently in 2006*) which I must admit now, may have been an irresponsible and hasty move or perhaps a stupid one when I think about it, I have had to work alone at motivating myself to fight the symptoms of FMS using mainly alternative therapies and treatments, but combining them with the conventional treatment of inflammatory tablets on the worst days.

Saying that, up to 2006 I have to admit that I did a pretty good job, despite my spontaneous decision to fight the fibromyalgia alone. I am no hippie or new age follower, but learning to channel the negative and painful energies using alternative therapies, then replacing them with positive energy has really helped me to personally cope with this condition and although using crystals, homoeopathy, meditation and other natural healing sources on their own have little effect, combining these alternative therapies and treatments with gentle exercise, a good vegetarian diet and self-discipline in my case has helped to reduce the effects of the various symptoms - *some of the time*. Some people even believe they have a guardian angel helping them along this rocky road of good and bad days, but whatever you believe in, finding the right balance to help you manage this condition is vitally important.

Now, I don't for one minute recommend that others suffering with fibromyalgia or any other similar type of condition follow my way of thinking, as the help and advice of someone medically qualified should be your first consideration, but I am the type of person that is not prepared to wait for others to sort out my fibromyalgia or osteoarthritis symptoms and will go out of my way to get things done in a battle to alleviate my own pain and discomfort... However, unlike many sufferers of these conditions, I am lucky enough not to suffer to the extremes of being unable to move without the aid of crutches, or the use of a wheel chair and that's the way I hope to remain.

Think positive – that's my motto!

<u>How I Manage My FMS</u>

As I do manage to get by on very little sleep and endure the pain, discomfort and times when I would rather not move, keeping motivated and happy on the lowest days is never easy. Not a single day goes by that I am free from a constant dull throbbing and often burning painful ache in my limbs of which my hips, knees, wrists, fingers and shoulders always seem to be the main areas to suffer, but I some how manage to re-channel the pain, discomfort and cope. Don't ask me how I do this as I don't know, but I put a lot of it down to daily meditation, and this doesn't mean I sit on the floor on a puffed up cushion with my legs crossed, chanting strange verses!

However, meditation is my way of relaxing and switching off from the symptoms, and just as a tip at this point if you do wish to have a go at meditating, then make sure you do this at a time during the day when you cannot be disturbed by the children, the husband, the dog or any household appliances. If necessary, evacuate the house of people for half an hour, turn off the television, unplug the telephone and put on some calming background music. I personally enjoy classical or commercially purchased mediation music CD's for relaxation, with my favourite being 'Lotus Morning' by James Harry from the "New Beginnings" series. However, the choice of music is yours as it is all down to personal taste. I know some people that meditate to the sounds of dolphins or the ocean, which are also extremely soothing. With meditating, you haven't got to sit on the floor. You can use a comfortable chair, settle down on your bed or soak in the bath (but don't fall asleep! Be sensible with this option) and then once you are comfortable, begin to think positive thoughts, whilst developing your breathing technique. By learning to channel negative energies away from your body and replacing them with the energy from all those positive thoughts you may find that relaxation and the breathing techniques come more naturally, enabling you to have some calm between the discomforts of FMS. So go on, be a devil and try it…

"If nothing else, it's nice to have some time to yourself"

I personally set myself daily targets of short sessions twice a day of either Gentle Yoga or Tai-chi which on those bad days often fails to go further than the warming up exercises, a few basic techniques and the warm down exercises. I enjoy walking everyday of which I am lucky enough to have a couple of paddocks for exercising not only my dogs and ponies, but myself 2-3 times daily which is ideal on the bad days as I am only a short distance away from the comfort of my house, or I can sit on the bench and take time out to regain some energy. This also enables me to walk at a distance and pace that I am happy with and something I have gradually worked up to.

"*Remember to always consult with your Doctor before attempting any form of exercise*"

I also enjoy cooking and eating a healthy well balanced vegetarian diet (I actually dislike the taste of meat and fish, although the concerns for animal welfare are also close to my heart). Having a positive and happy look on life undoubtedly play a huge part in how I deal with my fibromyalgia and osteoarthritis, and these are combined with many alternative therapies and supplements. Being happy, physically and mentally motivated helps you to live with fibromyalgia and other arthritic conditions. Being miserable and unmotivated will undoubtedly make you depressed and the symptoms will gradually become more and more unbearable as the condition worsens.

In writing this book on my own experiences, I hope that others with fibromyalgia or similar conditions will get inspiration and motivate themselves in to fighting their symptoms. Some people can naturally cope better with pain and discomfort more than others, and luckily I am one of those people. However, everyone needs to try and manage their own discomforts and what helps one person may not necessarily help another, so basically its trial and error. Self treating also means that whilst you are trying out different treatments your finances can suffer, but it is worth it if you can find a treatment that helps to alleviate some of the symptoms. As a person I make a stand on treating these symptoms using alternative treatments, which I will discuss later in this book. However, some alternative treatments work for me, but as we are all individual and we all suffer with various degrees of pain, discomfort and symptoms, then what helps me will not necessarily help you and I will emphasize at this point that I am not saying that what methods I choose to use are a miracle cure. They are certainly not, but they suit me and help with my own symptoms of fibromyalgia and osteoarthritis.

As already mentioned, I still use conventional medication like most people with this condition, but only when the symptoms are really bad as I prefer not to pump too many man made chemicals through my human system and I gave up on the prescription sleeping treatments, such as the anti-depressants a long time ago, but again some people naturally need more sleep than others and these treatments can help people to over come their sleep disorders. I prefer to use more natural therapies and treatments to help me sleep. These can include:

A good well balanced diet

Stress & Anxiety reducing therapies

Valerian – which can be very effective for insomnia

Natura Homoeopathic pills

St John's Wort – which can help relieve depression related disturbed sleep

5HTP – which has also been known to improve sleep disorders

Heat pads with added Lavender oil.

For the days that create stress from simple everyday life strains and my normal techniques of relaxing need a bit more of a boost, then I use a product called Natracalm Passiflora.

As a person, I always remain positive, happy and love to laugh, as I always say this is one of life's greatest healers. I motivate myself into doing tasks that I set myself and I am not happy until I achieve them. Each day I set my self a target and I increase on this as and when I can. I refuse to sit down and be lifeless and aim to remain active without creating further discomfort. I also work at keeping myself at a suitable weight, as obesity will place extra strains on the already painful points of the body and as an overweight person suffering with fibromyalgia or other arthritic conditions, the ability to keep active will be further reduced as well as encouraging other health concerns to develop. A little exercise is better than none at all and it really does make you feel good about yourself. I have found that an aerobic ball is very helpful and comfortable to use for gentle exercise and it certainly beats trying to exercise at floor level as getting down is hard enough, but getting back up another matter.

"Laughter is one of life's Greatest Healers"

I am no nutritionist, but common sense should tell you to *'Watch what you eat'*, by reducing your calorie intake. For example, if a recipe asks for two tablespoons of oil or sugar, then measure it. Pouring it straight from the bottle or sugar bag thinking you have the right amount will almost every time increase the amount that you should have used and undoubtedly an increase in fat and sugar will encourage weight gain. Rather than snacking on crisps and chocolate, replace it with healthy raw carrots, sesame seeds, pumpkin seeds and fresh fruit. Make yourself a tasty fruit or vegetable smoothie for breakfast as this can give you a good percentage of your daily requirements and an ideal alternative if like me, you find eating fruit tedious. If you can't be bothered to make your own, then you can buy a variety of smoothie flavours from health stores and supermarkets, but do pay attention to the nutritional information on the packaging to make sure that the product has no added sugar.

Experiment and find foods that you enjoy, then make them part of your meals. I find ordinary fruit like apples a real bore, but a bowl of fresh strawberries, cherries, apricots, raspberries, plums and gooseberries and I'm in heaven. Now that I pay more attention to what I do eat, I have found that I now eat a good variety of meals and because they are well balanced I know longer need to snack between meals, which means I have lost weight and now weigh a slim 9 stone, which is healthy for my height. At my heaviest I weighed an atrocious 11 ½ stone. My apologies, but I still prefer the old fashioned weights and measures. A family video shocked me into doing something about my weight, as I was horrified at my unflattering figure (*a bit like the back end of a buffalo*) and with the loss of weight the fibromyalgia is undoubtedly more manageable.

Drink plenty of water to flush out all those toxins, to prevent dehydration, and to maintain your body's natural balance. There is nothing wrong with drinking tap water, but if you prefer the taste of mineral water, then there are plenty of varieties to choose from. Try adding a squeeze of fresh lemon to your water, as it makes a nice refreshing drink.

I have recently started using *'Activated Liquid Zeolite'* , or the actual item that I'm taking is *'Znatural'* the original patented product as a way to help detoxify my body, as I personally believe that this can go along way to preventing a lot of illnesses. This product was developed from 14 years of research by Ohio biochemist Harvey Kaufman, and the invention sold to the biochemist Rik Deitsch (*1*) and described by health guru Dr. Gabriel Cousens as "an alchemical gift from God to help us face our present-day health challenges…"(*2*) Zeolites are a group of minerals formed when molten lava and ash from ancient volcanoes are mixed with sea water. These zeolites have been seen to remove heavy metals, toxins and other compounds from the body, whilst supporting a healthy immune system. Apparently it attracts and then buffers excess protons which cause acidity, which may then help with conditions such as arthritis. I have to say since taking this supplement I have felt a lot better in my self and certainly have more energy. However, 'Znatural' and 'Active Zeolite Liquid' are not cheap at around £30.00 for a small 15ml dropper bottle which contains about 300 drops. More information on these products can be located via the website links found in the resource section at the back of my book.

Also be aware of food intolerances, as these can also make you feel unwell. If you crave certain foods, then you may find that you are actually intolerant to them and by eating the same food on a daily basis you can in fact create food sensitivities, which can lead to digestive disorders, nutritional imbalances and weight gain to name a few conditions.(*3)*

Food intolerances can also be related to many health conditions, which include Asthma, **Arthritis**, Bloating, **Crohn's disease**, Constipation, Diarrhoea, Eczema, **Fibromyalgia** and **Irritable Bowel Syndrome (IBS)**, Lethargy, Migraines and tiredness.(*4)*

Now I'm not saying that you should cut out all the edible pleasures in life as we all need our comfort food, but use these as a positive treat. I still have my glass of red wine and eat my favourite foods, but I have adapted the meals so that they provide the necessary reduced calories and I never cook with salt. People seem so obsessed with adding salt to food. Just watch a TV chef and see how much salt they add to their dishes, it really does horrify me. Yet food seasoned with herbs and naturally strong flavoured foods such as, garlic taste wonderful and really doesn't need to be spoilt with added salt, apart from this many foods naturally contain salt so why add more!

I love chocolate and crisps, so I eat a small chocolate bar in replace of the standard size and make it last longer by putting it in the fridge so it takes longer to chew, but just as enjoyable. I now only ever buy low fat crisps that contain the salt separately in a small blue bag which is thrown away. Or for an even healthier option make your own by oven roasting some thinly sliced potato and sprinkle with herbs. Sweet potatoes make nice alternative to home made crisps. So it is possible to have the best of both worlds. For those of you that enjoy your meat, then simply cut down on the red meats and eat more white meat, such as chicken and add more fish into your diet. Grill or Steam as a healthier option and try to avoid eating too much junk food, such as burgers and chips. If you do want a burger and chips for a meal, then try oven roasted sweet potato chips and a spicy bean burger placed between a sesame seed bun with side salad. It's delicious and one the children will enjoy too. Apparently, eating a vegetarian or vegan diet can also help reduce the symptoms of fibromyalgia, so it certainly is well worth trying. However, this is something I will discuss further on in this book.

A couple of other points I would like to mention under this section, is that you should be aware of the effects of some foods. For example:

The Nightshade Family: There have been reports that some people may experience an increase in pain after consuming vegetables related to the nightshade family.

These include vegetables, such as:

Bell Peppers

Potatoes and Tomatoes.

Tomatoes are known to contain high level of glutamates, which are associated with creating muscle pain in a small number of people. So basically, pay attention to what you eat and identify any foods that seem to increase your pain levels so that you can avoid them in the future.

Candida Yeast Infections, can cause many generalized symptoms, including:

Dizziness

Fatigue

Lethargy

Migraine Headaches

Muscle Pain

Weakness

It can also be associated with: Acne, Bladder Inflammation, Constipation,

Diarrhoea, Eczema, Rectal Itching, Irritable Bowel Syndrome (IBS), Flatulence, Food Sensitivities, Menstrual and Premenstrual problems. As well as having mental and emotional affects, including Confusion, Depression, Insomnia, Irritability, the Inability to Concentrate and Memory Loss to name a few.

Yeast problems have also been related to auto-immune conditions, which include Arthritis, Lupus and Multiple Sclerosis.

There has even been research on the effects and association of Candida yeast infections, with fibromyalgia implying that sufferers have a high yeast imbalance. *(5)*

If you do suffer with this condition then avoid yeast-containing foods, such as:

Beer

Wine

Bread and Pastries

And mold containing / supporting foods, such as:

Mushrooms

Malt or foods containing malt

As a supplement to aid this condition, you can try Grapefruit seed extract, which is a natural antifungal agent. Essential Fatty Acids aid the biochemical process, especially by strengthening the immune system. Fish oil and flaxseeds are great sources of EFA's and taking Probiotics can boost your body's beneficial bacteria in the digestive tract, such as Superdophilus and Bifido Factor. Normal intestinal flora has sufficient lactobacillus to digest food, but those suffering with candidiasis often have an imbalance that these supplements will correct. Try some of the tasty probiotic yoghurts now available in health shops and supermarkets.

Far too many people still show very little regard for a well balanced diet and any advice on nutrition is often pushed aside. I personally think it is sad that in today's society, we all too often simply *"live to eat"* rather than the sensible approach of *"eating to live!"* Especially as many people who do choose a healthier diet by removing a large proportion of their dairy products, processed foods and red meat find that they experience a noticeable improvement in their health, physically and mentally.

Do you realize that most commercially produced livestock is injected with hormones to fatten them up, and treated with alarming amounts of antibiotics to keep them alive and disease free. If you must eat meat then consider a more healthy option and buy organically produced meat which I know is a little more expensive, but far healthier for you. Experience the flavours and versatility of raw fruits and vegetables, wild brown rice, beans, pulses, seeds, nuts, etc. Instead of a fatty milkshake, try a freshly made vegetable juice or fruit smoothie. By following a well balanced diet, you will provide your body with all the right nutrients so that your body cells can detoxify and function correctly. However, please do discuss changes in diet with your doctor or a nutritionist, and introduce yourself to any new diet gradually so that your body becomes accustomed to the change of foods.

One of my life's goals was to write a book. Well, this is my second publication, but my first on fibromyalgia. This is something that I am proud to have achieved and another tick on my list of things to do before I am too old and grumpy to be bothered. Further on in this book you will find out more about me and the things I hope to achieve. If nothing else, I hope that it will encourage you to set yourself some targets in life. It doesn't matter what they are, or how long it takes you to achieve them as long as you do and with a little help and support from those around you, it is possible and it gives you a great feeling inside.

How Do I Keep Myself Happy?

Well, this is certainly not an easy task to achieve at times, but worth the extra effort. If you are feeling low and depressed, then getting yourself a pick me up can be hard. Identify something that makes you smile and happy and use it in your bid to get positive and above that grey zone of misery. It doesn't matter what it is, from an old family movie or photo album to your favourite comedy. Whenever you feel down, bring out your pick me up and try and avoid getting too deep into a depression because once there it will be a nightmare of a journey to escape that feeling. I've been there and it is not pleasant and it certainly wasn't me or my personality in what I could only describe as a living hell. You try to comfort eat to make yourself feel better, the novelty soon wears off and you then feel guilty and even more depressed, the extra weight gained from the over indulgence of chocolate, biscuits and crisps aggravates the FMS further leaving you in more pain and discomfort, so you yet again turn to your comfort zone for help and a quick fix. It's a vicious circle that's hard to break. At my worst I would easily eat up to eight full fat packets of crisps a day, too many biscuits to even count and would snack on chocolate bars hidden away in my own private stash of comfort food goodies. Thankfully I have managed to free myself from my depression and the comfort eating and because I now have a happy, positive outlook on life and I motivate myself as well as battling to treat my own fibromyalgia and osteoarthritis, the urge to binge comfort eat no longer exists.

As a person pre and post depression, I would class myself as naturally bubbly, a bit like a bottle of champagne that's had the cork removed too fast and with a wicked sense of humour to match. I can laugh at the most unusual things, but that's me and not everyone fizzes as I do, and if there is nothing amusing occurring then I will create my own fun. I can also find laughter through other peoples misfortunes. I know that's terrible, but hey you have to laugh and see the funny side of life. My poor husband has been on the receiving end of my humour on several occasions. It's a good job he is not easily offended.

I also enjoy watching Jim Carrey movies with 'Liar Liar' being my favourite film, as well as Laurel & Hardy movies and the good old English Carry On films. These always make me laugh and brighten up even the most negative days, as do many of the older style comedy series such as Only Fools and Horses, Open All Hours and the Kenny Everett Show. Laughter really is one of the best treatments to help you cope with this condition… I never go a single day without at least one laugh or a giggle.

"It's a natural antidote that you just can not purchase in a bottle."

As already mentioned there is my husband. He is not only supportive, but makes me happy and we laugh regularly. If you have family and friends that understand and support you, then life can have many laughs and the journey of coping with fibromyalgia or any other arthritic condition can be made just that bit easier.

"Remember, having FMS doesn't just affect you, but your entire family too"

Learn to talk, as a lack of communication will undoubtedly encourage problems to develop and once bottled up, they will appear as an explosion of emotions when triggered at their most vulnerable point.

One of my main ways of remaining positive is through music. I just love to sing as it's one of the most natural ways of expressing yourself. I can't say if I am any good, but hey I don't care whether I am well tuned and in harmony with the music or tone deaf as they say. Singing makes me feel good and when you feel good you can tackle anything. Listening to the music of my favourite artists is a daily pursuit that's never missed. I know he's not every ones cup of tea, but Barry Manilow has a voice in a million, as well as being a talented musician and song writer. To start life as an ordinary guy, then end up as a popular talent having come years of ups and downs to me is a real inspiration and to see him in concert in Las Vegas is one of those items on my list of things to do. The Bee Gees, Country music, Shakira and most everyday music that has a decent beat will always bring a smile to my face, even on those not so good days and some decent classical music in the background is excellent for relaxing and meditating.

Another item on my list of things to do is to learn to play the piano. I was always interested with this amazing instrument at school, but unfortunately I only ever got as far as playing *'Three Blind Mice'* and my music teacher allocated me a trumpet instead, much to the horror of my parents who suffered the noise for well over two years before I got bored with the brass polishing. I think the piano will not only keep my motivation high, but will keep my fingers and ankles moving.

However, one point here that I must express is that any repetitive activity such as playing the piano, knitting, cross stitch, etc, can in fact exacerbate the problem so a little of these activities every day is better than trying to practice or knit for several hours a day.

My husband spoilt me with a new electric piano and now I practice in short sessions every couple of days. It will take me longer to learn, but that doesn't matter as I'm in no hurry. I love to make my own music inspired by my own daily moods. Learning the basic notes was easy, grasping the chords is another matter, but this is another target I will achieve. Several years ago I started to learn the electric lead guitar, but because of the weight placed on targeted areas from this instrument, I have found that these past few years it has started to create too much discomfort, so basically I decided to pluck my last string and have a go at something else. Anyway, I can't be that bad, as my dogs remain by my side when playing the piano, where as the guitar they would all dive for cover at the nearest and quietest place.

My beautiful Border Collies amuse me daily, as do the many dogs that pass by with their owner's as Acre Fen Canine Crèche guests, or up until recently people seeking behavioural advice for their dogs. I am a Canine Behaviour Consultant by profession with a certificate in Dog Psychology and the Canine Angels website is now only running for informational purposes. I no longer provide personal consultations, as I do find these can be physically and mentally demanding. Running my website advice pages also allows me to follow my interests by enabling me to do as much or as little a day, depending on how I feel. With Acre Fen Canine Crèche, I only accept well behaved/trained pets as the more demanding pets, especially the dogs would drain my energy levels and increase the pain and discomfort I deal with on a daily basis and again the hours are worked to suit me.

One thing fibromyalgia sufferers will understand is that having an understanding employer is hard to find, so getting and keeping a suitable job is never easy. This is why I prefer to be my own boss and if I need time out then I only have myself to answer to and because I am my own boss I allow myself at least two free days a week and one full week free of other peoples pets every month. On top of this I enjoy running my websites including 'Fibromyalgia and Arthritis' (previously known as Living With Fibromyalgia) of which there is a link at the back of this book under the resources section. I also established Hamster Rescue (UK), which provides mainly advice, but can take in a small number of old, unwanted and neglected hamsters. This is not a registered charity, but a small self-funded rescue doing its bit to help animals in need. There is something so relaxing about stroking an animal. It helps soothe those tense discomforts and places them at the back of your mind as the pleasure and positive experience takes over from simply communicating and handling a pet, whether it be a dog, cat, hamster or pony, they can all make such a difference to people's lives. Why on earth there are so many unwanted animals and so much animal cruelty in the world is heart breaking, but that's another story to be discussed another day.

Having my dogs and ponies provides me with the motivation to do a bit of exercise, even if this is just some basic grooming, as well as helping me to relax. My animal companions help me cope with my fibromyalgia and more recently my osteoarthritis in more ways than one.

Coping with this condition is not easy and can be a constant battle to keep motivated, especially on the bad days. Even the housework can be a chore, especially the ironing and vacuuming to simply cleaning out the bath, and turning the mattress on the bed. Thankfully this is one of the tasks that my husband now takes charge of. I have developed a routine by which I do the upstairs one day in the week and the downstairs on another day. Unless you have a really active household, then a house shouldn't need to be dusted and vacuumed on a daily basis and never allow it to get neglected, as keeping on top of the dust and clutter will be a nightmare. Ironing gets done when I only have a few items this way it is not so much of a task to complete.

Other family members should be encouraged to help, so make sure they clean the bath or shower out after them, get them to clean the windows, help with the bed making, vacuum the house or tidying the garden, etc. On a positive point, I have to say there's nothing better than a husband doing the washing up after a meal – who needs a dishwasher as a must have appliance... This is far more entertaining!

Having fibromyalgia means that you need to learn to plan your days according to how you feel and avoid pushing yourself too far as this will result in more discomfort than what the day started with. Make time for your self to relax, re-energize and allocate that all important happy hour of laughter every day.

Finally, remember to set your self targets and have something to aim for in life. Some of the other things I would like to do over the next few years, other than those already mentioned include:

1) Having a go at Clay Pigeon Shooting and Golf, if my bones and muscles don't get the better of me. It's also something my husband and I can enjoy together.

2) I would also like to travel and visit the American Cities of New York, Chicago, Las Vegas and Miami. The vibrant energy of these individual cities is fascinating and this vast country has so much for a person to see and experience and not just in the cities, but also their national parks and the outstanding scenery and wildlife that make up these natural treasures. Perhaps even have a go at western trail riding in Montana, which I believe would be a lovely way to explore natures finest.

3) One other place I would love to visit is the South American country, Peru where I would like to visit the lost cities of the Inca's. What an absolutely beautiful and colourful country to explore.

4) And perhaps even write and have a few more books published, as I thoroughly enjoy the challenge. I may even write a book on my experience of having Osteoarthritis in the future.

All these depend on how I manage both my fibromyalgia and osteoarthritis, but one thing I am determined to achieve is not to allow the symptoms to take over my life completely!

What exactly is Fibromyalgia

When I was diagnosed with fibromyalgia, I spent many hours researching this condition and trying to locate helpful resources. I was amazed that I could locate so much more information on fibromyalgia from other countries, such as the USA and Canada than what I could locate here in the United Kingdom. However, the few information resources that there are in the United Kingdom are good and offer some excellent information and support. Thankfully more and more information and support continues to be established, including many local help groups.

At the back of this book you will find an excellent resource section too many fibromyalgia and arthritis links from around the world that I have personally found to be a wealth of information. Now, let us proceed to the more descriptive section of this book.

Well what is Fibromyalgia?

The name Fibromyalgia is the term used to explain painful fibrotic changes in the soft body tissue/parts including the muscles, tendons and ligaments, but has come to mean much more to those of us that suffer from this syndrome. From my own experience and research, this is how I understand the condition.

Fibromyalgia, also known as FMS Syndrome and has only recently been used as a term to diagnose people that suffer from multiple abnormalities revolving around chronic musculoskeletal pain and irritation. The problem is that this condition has only been recognized during the past couple of decades and is still widely misunderstood, making diagnosis and treatment difficult. The diagnostic criteria was formulated by The American College of Rheumatology in 1990 (*6)* and despite increasing research into this condition, the etiology and pathophysiology of this syndrome is still poorly understood (*7)*. Fibromyalgia can affect anyone from the very young to the elderly, male and female, although women seem to be affected with this condition more than men. However, whether you are male or female the painful symptoms and the non-restorative sleep patterns are the same and living with this condition can be a real nightmare.

During the deep phase of sleep for 'non' sufferers of FMS, the immune functions and serotonin production occur to levels that allow people to function during the hours when they are awake. However, people with fibromyalgia suffer from a reduction of serotonin levels and an impaired immune function. People with this condition will also recognize the terminology 'Fibrofog' which is associated to cognitive problems, such as concentration and retention issues and the lack of short term memory, etc, and as pain levels increase, sleep is further disrupted leading to an increase in fibrofog.

Although, fibromyalgia is not life threatening, it does change your life drastically and living with it is no joy as many suffers will relate to. Finding help and support can also be a challenge as many people simply do not understand the pain sufferers are in as to most people they simply just look fatigued. It is only really close friends, family and the sufferer's medical consultants/doctors that understand the reality that surrounds our daily lives.

The cause of fibromyalgia is still unknown, but apparently there are five distinct areas which reappear in medical research. These are:

Toxicity:

Exposure to organic chemicals or pesticides

Trauma and Stress
Genetic Type

Immunologic - Viral or bacterial infection, or after immunisation

Post-Traumatic especially Cervical Spine compression, which is commonly located through whiplash accidents.

Low blood serum levels:

These are found in essential amino acids, including tryptophan. The tryptophan is then converted to serotonin in the brain. The serotonin is the chemical involved in sleep regulation, pain control, and immune system function.

Mineral imbalances:

Preliminary findings have indicated that red blood cell magnesium levels are low. The magnesium is an essential catalyst for producing energy at the cellular level and a lower concentration may contribute to symptoms of fatigue. Other minerals, such as zinc may also be abnormally low.

Abnormal muscle cell biochemistry may exist:

A reduction in energy stored in the muscles combined with a poor oxygen supply, have been found by one research team. It has been suggested that an enhanced susceptibility to muscle tissue injury may contribute to the pain of fibromyalgia.

Delta sleep anomaly that often occurs in FMS:

The impact of disturbed sleep can have a severe effect on the body's hormonal and immunological functions. Sleep disorders can be observed on an electroencephalogram (recorder chart) on which the brainwaves, characteristics of waking appear interspersed among the shallow rhythmic brain waves typically seen on an EEG recorder chart during deep sleep. Basically, when fibromyalgia patients wake up, they feel un-refreshed, which can be best described as though we had not slept at all.

Finding relief to FMS is also a challenge and takes a considerable amount of understanding, and understanding fibromyalgia goes a long way to helping cope with this syndrome and to living a half normal lifestyle. I personally set out to gain further knowledge on the condition so that I could help treat the symptoms myself rather than relying on others, such as the medical profession. Learning to help your self is an important part of coping with fibromyalgia.

While no pathological changes in the muscle tissues have been demonstrated on any type of examinations and routine laboratory tests usually reveal no abnormalities, fibromyalgia sufferers will demonstrate very tender muscular points which cause a great deal of pain. Diagnosis is part formed from a person having at least 11 – 18 tender points, which are located around the body from the knees to the hips, elbows, chest, shoulders and neck, etc. Fibromyalgia is often referred to as the arthritis of the soft body tissues, where as normal arthritis affects the bones.

Various, research on this condition as indicated that people with fibromyalgia are low in growth hormones, which help to repair the body's muscle tissue. They have also shown a decrease in the blood flow to certain areas of the brain. One of these areas is known as the thalamus, which helps to control hormone levels. Sufferers have also been found to have up to three times the normal human level of the neurochemical 'Substance P', which is located in the spinal fluid and determines the pain level that the person is experiencing. It has been found that the chemical component of fibromyalgia has been identified to be a reduction in serotonin, but an increase in the Substance P.

Fibromyalgia also has two category types. Primary Fibromylagia is diagnosed when no other diagnosable conditions are found, whereas Secondary Fibromyalgia is diagnosed as a result of other recognised health conditions including, Arthritis, Lupus and Multiple Sclerosis to name a few.

Nothing about fibromyalgia is normal and it never follows a set course. On good days, sufferers are tempted to over exert themselves, leading to a weakened energy and immune system. However, on the bad days, sufferers can be tempted not to move about, further increasing the risk of stiffness, pain and/or discomfort. Finding the correct balance certainly is not easy.

I along with other people who suffer with fibromyalgia can suffer a whole host of other physical symptoms including, but not limited to:

Chest Pain

Constipation

Depression

Diarrhoea

Disturbed Sleep

Extreme Fatigue

Headaches

Muscle Pain and/or discomfort

Insomnia

I will discuss the many related symptoms in more detail in the chapter 'Fibromyalgia Symptoms' later in this book.

It can also be difficult describing this condition, as every individual sufferer has different symptoms and pain levels. However, sufferers will all commonly have aches and pains similar to those related to flu, exhaustion, sleeplessness, stiffness, tenderness, joint pain and/or discomfort, but unlike flu, our symptoms don't fade away, but remain day in and day out throughout the years.

Our human bodies are full of nerve sensors which allow us to feel pain, cold, heat, touch, smell, taste, etc. Unfortunately, with fibromyalgia these sensors transmit the various signals as pain ranging from a tingling sensation, burning sensation to severe muscle and joint pain. It can be so severe that even wearing certain clothes, opening jars and cans, or being touched can be painful. Other tasks that I find difficult at times include, holding an umbrella, lifting the kettle or teapot and even wearing a watch is uncomfortable at times. It's amazing how simple, everyday items and chores can create so much discomfort and pain.

So, fibromyalgia simply means pain of the muscle fibers. However, it is more correctly defined as a connective tissue disorder. Every cell in our human body is surrounded by connective tissues, including the muscles and nerves and the chronic tension that is related to FMS affects the body's connective tissues. So basically, when our bodies suffer trauma through injury for example, the connective tissues become inflamed resulting in pain.

Fibromyalgia has also been referred to as a "chronic invisible illness", and it isn't just a form of muscular rheumatism. It's a whole host of conditions which can be related to neurotransmitter dysfunction, etc.

At the moment there is no treatment that can completely resolve fibromyalgia, although researchers are working on this. However, there are many treatments that can help to alleviate the pain and discomfort. The problem is, finding the treatment that suits and provides the individual sufferer the best relief. Trigger points can be relieved by some types of physical therapy. However, it does take commitment on the part of any fibro sufferer to understand good nutrition, follow a program of gentle stretching and moderate exercise, and being sensible in recognizing their own limitations. Finding the perfect balance, so that the quality of life is good, is not easy. I will discuss the various treatments later in this book, including the ones I have used in the past and presently.

Some physicians have speculated that fibromyalgia begins with the Mononucleosis virus, and followed by the lingering Epstein's bar virus. It has also been suggested that many fibromyalgia sufferers have had a recent heavy emotional or physical trauma prior to the onset of FMS and that illness and hormone changes can all play a part in this condition, as well as sufferers failing to fall in to the deepest phase of sleep. As previously mentioned earlier in this book, this is known as the 'Delta Stage' or 'Non-restorative Sleep', which prevents the muscles shutting down, then resting and repairing properly. It is also possible that a combination of these symptoms in a person may develop into fibromyalgia.

Also mentioned in the beginning of my book, Doctors seem in disagreement about any hereditary link, but some do believe that when fibromyalgia runs in families that an inherent predisposition may be present. This is the one option I would really like to see more research into, as I personally believe that there has too be some sort of hereditary link. It surely can not be coincidence that several members of one family can suffer with fibromyalgia, arthritis, rheumatism, etc...

As for the research into fibromyalgia there have been some interesting studies highlighting the effects of food on the symptoms of rheumatic conditions and the possible benefits of vegetarian food, but unfortunately most of them have only involved rheumatoid arthritis so very little information on the effects for those with fibromyalgia are available. However, some studies have indicated that diet plays a role in fibromyalgia *(8)*, with certain foods apparently aggravating the condition. These foods included meat, wine/alcohol, coffee, chocolate, sugar and some fruits such as apples and citrus fruits. Another small study by Hostmark *Et Al* *(9)* revealed an increased subjective well-being among some fibromyalgia sufferers after they had been on a vegetarian diet for three weeks, although this particular study was actually implemented to investigate other research. Another recent study evaluated the effects of a strict vegan diet on the symptoms of fibromyalgia resulted in the vegan diet alleviating the fibromyalgia symptoms short term *(10)* and further studies have now been recommended including the effectiveness of a vegan diet in the long term. Studies have shown that a vegan diet can improve symptoms of this condition. One such study on a Finnish group of sufferers put on a vegan diet found that the animal-free diet alleviated the symptoms of fibromyalgia including pain, morning stiffness and high urinary sodium levels. The study also showed that the patients that were on the vegan diet had lower cholesterol levels, reduced weight and were able to sleep better than those not on a vegan diet.

So there you have it. A brief description on '*What is Fibromyalgia?*' and how research is progressing to find that all important treatment that will bring relief to so many sufferers around the world. Allowing non-sufferers of fibromyalgia to read this book, whether they are family members, friends or work colleagues may help them understand this condition a little better, so that they can be more supportive, especially on those negative days where the discomfort is at its worst.

"A friend is a close companion on rainy days, someone to share with through every phase…
Forgiving and helping to bring out the best, believing the good and forgetting the rest."

How To Diagnose Fibromyalgia

The only people that are fully qualified to diagnose fibromyalgia are those professionals in the medical world, such as GP's and Consultant Rheumatologists, and it can be a long process of elimination of other ailments before diagnosing FMS.

Physical therapists, nurses and other health care professionals may suggest that your symptoms are similar to fibromyalgia, but the symptoms may also be the warning signs of other health conditions.

Your Doctor should perform various tests to rule out other similar causes of discomfort and symptoms.

These should include:

Arthritis, including Degenerative Arthritis, Rheumatoid Arthritis and Osteoarthritis

ME

Lupus

Raynauds Disease

If these come back normal then you should be referred to a Rheumatology consultant for further tests.

With fibromyalgia the muscles are usually extremely painful and quite localised. These are known as "trigger" or "tender" points, which when pressed even very gently may cause excruciating discomfort and pain. Fibromyalgia is the second most common rheumatological condition after osteoarthritis.

Fibromyalgia is often associated with a whole range of other symptoms and not just the muscle pain, as explained in this book. Fibromyalgia also has a considerable overlap with chronic fatigue syndrome, or ME. However, the main difference is the very severe nature of the muscular pains in fibromyalgia.

"The Tender points must be considered 'Painful', not just tender to touch."

Unfortunately, at the moment there isn't a single blood test or x-ray that will diagnose fibromyalgia. However, this condition can often begin with trauma, such as a car accident or a fall. Someone who is generally a bit stiff/achy and is at the same time experiencing a lot of stress may suddenly find that they fail to recover from the injury and that their muscle pain goes on getting increasingly worse. All the blood tests done by various doctors and specialists will tend to be normal and quite often, both the doctors and patients are confused. The diagnosis is, therefore exclusively made on the basis of the way the symptoms are localised (Trigger points), of which sufferers usually have between 11 and 18 areas of pain and/or discomfort in all four quadrants of their body.

For example:

1) Are there enough tender points in the muscles of all four limbs?

2) Has the pain been present for a minimum duration of 3 months?

3) Is the tenderness/pain present in at least 11 of the 18 specified tender points when pressure is applied?

4) Are all the conventional tests normal?

5) Is the clinical history consistent with increasing, unexplained and very severe muscle pain?

Drawing the human body was never my best topic of art and this image is no exception. Fibro-Fleur as I've nicknamed her does look a little animated, sorry for herself, and probably has the worst drawn legs in history. However, she does highlight the main target areas of localized pain.

Diagram Displaying the Trigger (Tender) points:

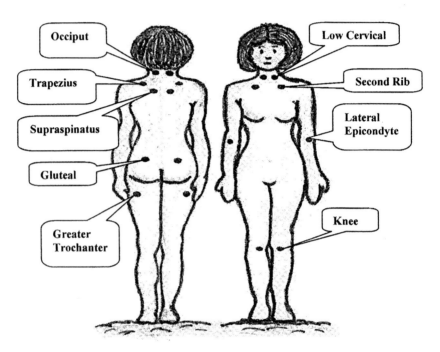

Occiput

Low Cervical

Trapezius

Second Rib

Supraspinatus

Lateral Epicondyte

Gluteal

Greater Trochanter

Knee

AJC Fibro Trigger Points Image © 2007 All Rights Reserved

I must mention at this point that some sufferers, including myself can experience more tender points, and endure days when our pain levels are so high that it feels like every part of our body is in pain.

Basically, a diagnosis is therefore based on listening carefully to the person's history, while conducting a careful examination of their muscles, bones and joints. A family history of arthritic conditions may also be taken into account.

On the whole fibromyalgia is a very difficult condition to treat. There are several approaches used in complementary medicine that may be of help to people with fibromyalgia and some alternative therapies may also be beneficial.

Fibromyalgia Symptoms

Like many people with FMS, I personally suffer from a combination of several symptoms, of which some are worse than others. I have marked some of these in the list below with a *, although there are others that could be highlighted. Fibromyalgia is not a disease, but this condition can cause major disruption to daily life and is not just irritating, but unpleasant.

Pain, Tiredness and Sleep Disturbance are the main symptoms of Fibromyalgia - Most people feel the pain of fibromyalgia as, Aching, Stiffness and Tiredness in the muscles, tendons and ligaments around joints. It may feel worse first thing in the morning or as the day goes on, or with activity. It may affect one part of the body or several different areas such as the limbs, neck or back.

Fatigue (tiredness) may be the most severe aspect of fibromyalgia - There may be overall Tiredness and a Lack of Energy, and/or Muscle Fatigue as well as a Lack of Endurance.

Either way, it can be difficult to climb the stairs, do the household chores, or go shopping – let alone go to work. Becoming less fit may also make matters worse.

Here are some other symptoms/conditions that Fibromyalgia sufferers can develop.

It's quite a list, and by no means complete:

*Tingling, Numbness, *Clumsiness
*Poor Circulation / Swelling of the Hands and/or Feet, Poor Co-ordination
*Joint Pain, *Bruising, *Muscle Spasms, *Pelvic Pain and *Chest Wall Pain
*Skin Itching and/or Rashes, *Allergies
*Headaches/Migraine, *Irritability, *Feeling low or weepy and Neurological Symptoms*

Dizziness, Anxiety, Confusion, *Mood Swings, Memory Loss and Panic Attacks
Speech Problems, such as mixing up words
*Forgetfulness, *Poor Concentration
*Sensitivity to the cold, noise, bright lights, etc, *Cold hands and/or feet
Needing to pass water, or feeling an urgent need to pass water
*Painful and Irregular Periods and/or PMT
Lack of Endurance
Irritable Bowel Syndrome, Interstitial Cystitis (Inflammatory disorder affecting the walls of the bladder
Raynaud's Disease
Cognitive Problems
Hearing Problems
*Waking up feeling un-refreshed
Anxiety and/or Depression
Hypoglycemia
Mitre Valve Prolapse
Gastro-Esophageal Reflux Distrophy (GERD)
Hypothyroidism
Chronic Fatigue Syndrome (CFIDS, CFS)
Vertigo
Temporomandibular Joint Disorder (TMJ)
Myofascial Pain Syndrome (MPS)
Carpel Tunnel Syndrome
Costochondritis
Sleep Apnea
Fever
Lupus
*Osteoarthritis (Diagnosed 2006) and Rheumatoid Arthritis.
Multiple Chemical Sensitivity (MPS)
Polymyalgia Rheumatica
Seasonal Affective Disorder (SAD)
Sjogren's Syndrome
*Sore Throats, Swollen Lymph Nodes and Mouth Sores
Sexual Dysfunction including painful intercourse for women and

impotence in men
*Eating Disorders, such as Anorexia, Bulimia, Food Bingeing, etc,
Digestive Problems and Weight Gain
Candidas (Yeast Infections)
Hair Problems, such as thinning/loss of hair and Nail Problems
Immune System Weakness or Immune Dysfunction
ADHD (Attention Deficit Hyperactivity Disorder)
Gulf War Syndrome (GWS) and Post Polio Syndrome

Please Note: Naturally symptoms like these can have other causes, and your doctor can help decide whether any further tests or advice is required. The severity of the symptoms in fibromyalgia can vary considerably and sufferers have a variety of different symptoms. There is a range from severe disruption of life to almost normal, and this spread causes problems in diagnosing the condition and can lead to varying medical opinions.

Health conditions having similar symptoms:

Lyme Disease - This disease is caused by a tick bite and symptoms are very similar to FMS and CFIDS. However, there is a test that can determine if you have Lyme disease, although some researchers are concerned that the test can give a false negative result. Your doctor will be able to provide plenty of information as will the internet.

Tension Myositis Syndrome - This condition can cause (or imitate) FMS and occurs when the muscles tense up under stress. Some people can get their whole body in a spasm of pain from getting stressed out emotionally. This condition can be helped by avoiding stress, using magnesium for muscle relaxation, taking warm baths or having a massage.

Thyroid - Symptoms of either hypothyroidism or hyperthyroidism can also be very similar to FMS. For example, with '*hypothyroidism*' the symptoms include fatigue, inability to tolerate cold, fertility problems, muscle weakness, muscle cramps, hair loss, recurrent infections, constipation, depression, difficulty concentrating and slow speech, etc. With '*hyperthyroidism*', the symptoms can include nervousness, irritability, a constant feeling of being hot, insomnia, fatigue, hair loss, hand tremors and a rapid heartbeat, etc. Blood tests can detect an under active or overactive thyroid gland and your doctor will be able to provide plenty of information on these conditions. Other health conditions that can display similar symptoms include:

Other conditions which can have similar symptoms include:

Ankylosing Spondylitis - Auto immune disease
Arthritic conditions – Rheumatoid Arthritis, Osteoarthritis and Degenerative Arthritis
Bacterial infections
Chronic Fatigue Syndrome
Lupus erythematosis - chronic inflammatory and auto-immune condition
Neurological diseases - Multiple Sclerosis, Neuropathy
Overuse and tempero-mandibular joint syndromes
Osteoporosis
Polymyalgia Rheumatica - Usually affects the elderly
Polymositis -inflamation and weakness in the voluntary muscles
Psychogenic Rheuamtisms - Emotional/psychological somatic disorder
Sjogren's syndrome - Rheumatic condition
Viral infections

Alternative Remedies

Fibromyalgia is frequently treated with prescription medications for muscle relaxants, analgesics, anti-depressants and/or sleeping tablets. However, more often these days, people suffering with FMS are referred to alternative therapy clinics for Massage Therapy, Acupuncture, Yoga, Biofeedback and other natural treatments. Although, not one single treatment, whether alternative or conventional can cure this condition they can certainly help, either singularly or as a combination. I personally have found certain alternative treatments to be of benefit.

Fibromyalgia is a condition that is always there. However, a flare-up can be triggered by infection, mental or physical stress, too much exercise, pregnancy, a motor vehicle accident, and even changes in the weather. When my pain gets to be too much, I try soaking in a tub of warm to hot water (a spar bath is lovely and relaxing and relatively cheap to purchase) and both alternatives will help to reduce the pain. However, where possible avoid completely giving up the exercise, as you may find that you feel even worse the next day.

Do Not Mope About... Exercise such as walking, gentle aerobics, gentle yoga, tai-chi, swimming, etc, can all help in keeping you mobile. Exercise will improve your blood flow and the oxygen to your muscles, which will help to prevent muscle pain. Remember, that with any form of exercise you need to do '**Warming Up** and **Cooling Down**' exercises to prevent muscle cramps. Set your self a target each day, but do not over do it.

Research has confirmed that exercise can be beneficial to those suffering from Fibromyalgia increasing the overall level of fitness. It can also help you to cope with pain and stress more effectively. Any form of gentle exercise, practiced regularly will help you to keep fit.

Endurance exercise aims to strengthen your heart and make your lungs more efficient. Some of the most beneficial endurance exercises for people with fibromyalgia are walking, exercising in water and using a stationary bicycle.

Tips for Safe Exercise

As already mentioned you should always warm up and cool down. After the warm up exercises you should gradually increase the intensity of your exercise programme to help prevent injuries. Do your chosen activity at a moderate rate so that your breathing and heart rate are mildly increased, and you feel warmer. If your pain increases – stop exercising immediately, but do try and finish with the cool down techniques. You should wear comfortable, loose fitting clothes and shed layers to adapt to increases in temperature. Wear non-slip shoes, which should also be shock-absorbent and provide good support. Remember, by implementing cooling down exercises you will allow your body to naturally return to its normal pace and help to prevent injury.

Stretching and Strengthening Exercises.

Exercise such as gentle yoga, tai-chi and swimming are beneficial because they reduce stiffness and help keep your muscles strong and joints flexible. When swimming to try and use a swimming pool that is a warm temperature.

What is Tai Chi?

Tai Chi Chuan, or taijiquan, is an ancient Chinese form of co-ordinated body movements focusing on the cultivation of internal energy 'chi' or 'qi'. Its aim is to harmonise the mind, body and spirit, promoting both mental and physical well-being through softness and relaxation. When practiced correctly the movements of tai chi appear rhythmical, effortless and in continuous flow. It gently tones and strengthens your muscles and improves your balance and posture. It can also be of benefit to some medical conditions, such as cardiovascular, respiratory and digestive disorders. I have found it to be a great benefit to my own FMS.

With practice you can become revitalised, relaxed, tolerant, self-confident and stronger and healthier in both mind and body. Unlike most forms of exercise and sport, tai-chi does not rely on strength, force and speed, making it ideal for people of both sexes, young and old alike whether strong or weak. It is this approach that makes tai chi such a unique form of exercise that brings benefits in many areas.

What is Yoga?

Yoga is a time-honoured practice for healing and sustaining the body, mind and spirit. It helps alleviate many symptoms of chronic illness such as anxiety, headaches and muscle tension while building strength, flexibility and stamina. Neither the illness, disability or, inexperience need prohibit one from enjoying these benefits. Yoga may be modified to meet the needs of all, as it is non-competitive and arises from within. It brings balance and harmony to the mind, body and spirit and an exploration of movement and breath. Yoga is powerful medium for individual healing.

By learning the skills of yoga, you will be able to reduce the negative effects of illness while improving the quality of your life. You can experience an integration of yoga and mindfulness-based stress management, as well as learn to listen to your pain and understand its meaning and message. With daily practice, you will find yoga becomes more natural and in the process learn the art of these techniques.

Deep Breathing

Gentle Stretches

Meditation

Restorative Postures

Somatic Awareness

Setting Limits and Boundaries

Again, yoga is something I find very helpful and it really does help to relax my own painful aches.

Emu Oil:

This is something I use to help soothe painful aches, and the particular gel I purchase also contains Glucosamine. Emu oil has natural anti-inflammatory properties and contains a high level of Linoleic acid, which is a substance associated with the smooth running of muscles and joints. Apparently, the Aboriginal tribesmen and Bushmen of Australia have used this ointment to aid soothing and healing. It is quite strong smelling, a bit like the product Deep Heat.

T.E.N.S Home Clinic:

This is something that I do find beneficial as pain relief and use regularly. Transcutaneous Electrical Nerve Stimulation (T.E.N.S) is a recommended aid to pain relief which is used in hospitals and clinics throughout the UK and is now available as a small personal unit for use in the home. It works by eliminating the pain by transmitting tiny electrical messages to the nerve endings. This produces 'Endorphins' which are the body's natural pain killers and provides a soothing relief from various types of pain including, back pain, rheumatic, joint and muscle pain. I paid £30 for my and its well worth it.

Dietary and Nutritional Supplements:

Make sure you have a well-balanced diet to receive all the necessary natural nutrients required. If, for whatever reason this is not possible, then take a vitamin and mineral supplement.

It is also recommended that you include 'Fresh Chives' and 'Nettles' in your diet, as these are high in Iron and Vitamin C, and also to increase your dietary intake of Magnesium.

Limit consumption of refined sugar, salt, red meat, dairy products, alcohol, coffee, tea and chocolate, and the intake of fats, especially saturated cooked processed fats and hydrogenated vegetables oils. Substitute these with cold pressed unprocessed vegetable oils.

Decrease or eliminate use of tobacco, as tobacco interferes with utilization of oxygen.

Increase your intake of whole grains, legumes, green leafy vegetables and fresh fruits, and also fish and poultry if you are a meat eater.

As already mentioned, I eat a vegetarian diet which I believe is a healthier option. Others recommend a Gluten or Wheat free diet. However, a recent research has been made on the benefits of a vegan diet, which apparently helps to alleviate FMS symptoms.

Glucosamine Hi-Strength with and without Chondroitin:

I take vegetarian Glucosamine and have found it to be fairly beneficial and would recommend that other sufferers give it a try. However, the vegetarian supplement is only available in tablet form at present, but non-vegetarian versions are widely available. This treatment helps to maintain the □Connective Tissues' and 'Joints', which are continuously regenerating. You can purchase this supplement with added 'Vitamin C', or as I do take it separately. Vitamin C is an effective 'Anti-Oxidant' that is known for its role in tissue integrity. Calcium (Carbonbate) aids the strengthening of bones around the tendons, cartilage and ligaments. For those that choose to combine the 'Chondroitin', this is a constituent of the connective body tissues. This is available in tablet or liquid form, of which I personally think the liquid, is a better option as it gets into your system faster. You can purchase it without prescription from most reputable health food stores, but do shop around as the prices can vary considerably.

Some FMS sufferers have found that 'MSM' (*Methyl-Sulfonyl-Methane*) has helped and it's natural too. Further more, this is not a new product, but I for one had not heard of it until recently. The MSM works like an anti-inflammatory, where as the Glucosamine puts a lubrication back into the joints. Like all treatments, it will not work for everyone, but it is worth a try.

Herbalism:

Herbalism is an ancient form of medicine that uses plants and herbs to heal and many of today's drugs are derived from plants. For example, Aspirin originates from willows and morphine from poppies. These natural remedies can help many conditions ranging from allergies, hormonal problems to digestive complaints. For many people in the world, it is the only form of medicine available to them. Medical herbalists believe that the body has the capacity to protect and heal itself, and their job is to help the body to do this. However, there is a big difference between the substances used in conventional medicine and preparations dispensed by herbalists. In conventional medicine, scientists attempt to isolate what they term the active ingredients of a plant, whereas herbalists will use the whole of the relevant part of the plant, including the leaves, roots, etc.

However, herbal remedies can be very powerful, so you should discuss them with your doctor, especially if you are pregnant, taking any other medicines, or have a pre-existing medical condition, such as heart disease.

Beneficial Herbs/Natural Remedies:

Many of these are arthritis remedies, but may be beneficial for FMS symptoms.

Please remember – I am no herbalist and these are only printed as reference, so before taking any Alternative/Natural Remedies please do check with your Medical Practitioner first. This is because in some cases, herbal products can interact negatively with other medications, and these interactions can be dangerous. Herbal Remedies are 'Not' regulated, nor their quality controlled and despite many information resources circulating on herbs and their benefits, there is much to be scientifically proven. It is vitally important that you tell your doctor or pharmacist of any natural treatments you are taking, just the same as telling them about the conventional medications you use. These people are there to help and advise on what treatments are best used, especially when mixing medications.

Example of beneficial natural remedies:

Devils Claw – Traditionally used to treat pain. This is a natural anti-inflammatory, which may aid symptoms of Arthritis and Rheumatism.

Feverfew – A natural garden herb which has anti-inflammatory properties.

Rhus Tox – Homoeopathy remedy.

Celery – May help reduce the degeneration of joints.

Green Lipped Mussel – This may help reduce joint pain, improve flexibility and rebuild cartilage, and is a popular remedy for arthritic conditions.

Hemp Oil – Provides a good natural source of Omega 3 & 6 fatty acids, and a popular treatment for Rheumatoid Arthritis.

Yucca – A natural anti-inflammatory which may help alleviate symptoms associated to Arthritis, Osteoporosis and Rheumatoid Arthritis. This remedy contains many useful minerals including calcium and potassium.

Wild Yam – A natural anti-inflammatory and may help to regulate female hormone imbalances.

Stinging Nettle – A natural detox and tonic remedy which may be beneficial for Rheumatism and Arthritis.

Starflower Oil – Rich in Gamma Linolenic Acid, and may help reduce inflammation associated to Rheumatoid Arthritis.

St John's Wort – May help to improve serotonin levels and used as a natural anti-depressant.

SAMe – May reduce pain and inflammation associated with arthritis.

Royal Jelly – Traditional remedy used to treat Rheumatoid Arthritis. It may also be beneficial for insomnia and fatigue.

Omega-3, 6 & 9 – Essential fatty acids (EFA's) responsible for cell regeneration and health. May be beneficial for Arthritis and Depression.

Other Beneficial Herbs:

Angelica (Dong Quai), Astragalus, Echinacea, Garlic & Ginger: These all have immune enhancing properties.

Burdock: This helps to soothe pain related to arthritis, rheumatism and back ache.

Cayenne (Capsicum) Pepper: This relieves muscle pain when applied externally.

Chaparral: This helps to relieve leg cramps.

Crampbark: This is believed to be a natural muscle relaxant.

Dandelion: This can be effective in relieving inflammation and joint stiffness.

Passion Flower: This is believed to be an antispasmodic that can aid sleep.

Red Clover Tea: This is a general herb that can improve overall health and is believed to relax the body.

Turmeric and White Willow Bark: These are believed to have anti-inflammatory properties and may be useful for swelling and pain in joints.

Alfalfa, Horsetail, Oat Straw, Panax Ginseng, Papaya, Slippery Elm and Star Anise, may also be beneficial in relieving symptoms.

Visiting a qualified herbalist may have some benefits, so worth consideration.

Aromatheraphy – This is another therapy that the ancient Chinese, Egyptians, Greeks and Romans recognized as having therapeutic properties and they widely used essential oils and plant extracts. Modern aromatherapy is a result of the work researched by the two Frenchmen, Rene-Maurice Gatefosse, who discovered that Lavender oil quickly healed his own burnt hand and researched the healing qualities of plant oils. Dr Jean Valnet researched further during the Second World War whilst employed as a field surgeon. During this period of war, medical supplies were in short supply so Dr Jean Valnet used essential oils as an alternative and discovered that they had antiseptic, regenerative and healing properties, which were effective in treating the wounded soldiers.

Massage with Essential Oils can be beneficial:

Massage can help to alleviate the pain and discomfort associated with fibromyalgia, and by introducing essential oils in to the massage programme, can provide further benefits. These two essential oils I personally have found beneficial.

Helichrysum: This rich aromatic essential oil derives from the flower petals of the plant Helichrysum augustifolium. It can provide a soothing effect on your body and raises a person's natural spirit. This essential oil can be massaged into sore tissues where it can be beneficial in soothing away aches, pains, sprains and strains. It can also help relax a person's body and ease the tension and pain of tendons and muscles. Helichrysum can also be detoxifying, anti-allergenic, anti-inflammatory, analgesic, antibacterial, antiviral, astringent, expectorant, calming, warming and memory enhancing. In my personal experience a real good all round essential oil.

Lavender: This is another one of my personal favourites, and is distilled from the flowering tops of Lavender plants. Lavender is gentle to use and known to reduce soreness and sprains, and its scent is one of the best natural aromas to help induce sleep. Lavender can be applied on the temples or the back of the neck to help you relax. Or by mixing Lavender with Helichrysum, can help to relax painful muscles. Lavender is probably the most-used, and most often adulterated, essential oil in the world. Some of the effects of Lavender on the human body include, being a natural antiseptic, anti-spasmodic, analgesic, and anti-depressant, deodorant, diuretic, insect repellent, sedative and tonic.

These essential oils should always be combined with either massage lotion or almond oil. One part of each of the essential oils (two drops of each) to two parts massage lotion (or one squirt) or almond oil (12 drops). This mixture can be rubbed into a persons painful skin tissues and can provide relief.

However a word of warning, essential oils, by themselves, should never be applied directly to the skin. They are very concentrated and should be diluted with massage lotion before use.

Other Beneficial Essential Oils include:

Bergamot, Cedarwood and Chamomile - Used for Environmental Stress

Lavender, Patchouli and Sandlewood - Used for Mental Stress

Cardamom, Rose and Sandlewood - Used for Emotional Stress

Lemon, Patchouli and Rosemary - Used for Chemical Stress

Chamomile, Geranium and Lavender - Used for Physical Stress

It is recommended: That you consult a qualified aromatherapist before using essential oils, especially if you are pregnant or have high blood pressure, epilepsy, severe allergic responses or asthma. Never apply essential oils directly onto the skin - always combine with base oil, such as massage lotion or almond oil. Avoid accidental ingestion and 'Keep out of reach of children and pets!'

Other Alternatives Treatments to try:

Magnets: Some say they work others not. I personally have found that most of the versions I have tried provide very little help.

However, I do wear a:

Copper & Hematite combined bracelet: which I must admit does provide a warming sensation and my wrists definitely ache more without it being worn.

Copper and the effects of magnetism have been used for centuries to help alleviate pain and reduce inflammation in joints and by combining the therapeutic properties of copper and the gentle magnetic element of hematite has proven to be beneficial in my own experience.

Acupuncture: This is a traditional medicine which originated in China. It is at least 400 years old and is based upon a natural philosophy of harmonising the body with the elements found in nature. It is known to balance the emotional, mental and spiritual energies of the human body.

By inserting fine acupuncture needles at various sites on the body, the acupuncturist can alter blocked energy, eliminate pain and stimulate the body's own immune system, thereby encouraging self healing and preventing future disease. Primary diagnosis is by the taking of 12 pulses on the wrist and tongue examination.

Acupuncture treats all conditions by treating the person, not the disease, the cause not the symptom. It is a natural form of medicine, which has no side effects or harmful reactions. It is also relatively pain free.

Again some say it works, others not. I have tried this and found that is only beneficial as a short term relief. One thing, if you are squeamish over needles, then this one is probably best avoided as you will look like a pin cushion, although I personally didn't find the process of inserting the pins uncomfortable.

Hypnosis or Relaxation Therapy: As already mentioned earlier in this book, I have found that meditating can be extremely relaxing and beneficial in helping to cope with the symptoms of my own fibromyalgia.

As for the hypnosis, I can't comment as I have not yet travelled this road and personally, I am a little wary of this form of alternative therapy. However, other sufferers have found it to be helpful with their own symptoms.

Chiropractic: Again, this is something I have yet to try, but others have found it to be beneficial.

This therapy specializes in spinal manipulation with its emphasis on the skeleton and muscle alignment. Manipulation is the application of pressure, body leverage and physical thrust to a joint, or a group of related joints to restore proper alignment and function. A Chiropractor can provide relief from symptoms, improve joint and muscle function and speed up the recovery process. This is done without the use of excessive drug therapy and for some ailments, without the use of invasive surgery.

Bath Spa's & Jacuzzi's: I have personally found that a bath spa is beneficial in reducing my discomfort and for helping me to relax. These can be purchased at reasonable prices, depending on what type you choose, although the non-permanent versions will not keep your water at a set temperature. However, if you want a more luxurious permanent fixture then you can by commercially made baths with built in spa facility or go that extra mile and treat yourself to a Jacuzzi. These can be beneficial to various ailments and conditions as the constant thermostatically controlled heating system keeps optimum temperature, as the controllable flow of bubbles gently massages the body's tender, aching and bruised areas, providing relaxation and relief.

Hydrotherapy - The basic definition is the use of water, externally or internally, as a health treatment, and covers a wide variety of methods.

Internal use: This could be as simple as drinking water, or to the other extreme of being used in colon therapy.

External hydrotherapy: This covers many different methods, including:

1) Cold or Warm compresses, of which one particular treatment involves applying cold compresses which are warmed up naturally by the body. This reaction effects blood circulation, nerve activity and the body's muscles and tissues.

2) Soaking in the bath.

3) Specialized equipment, such as whirlpool baths.

4) Water-based (pool) exercise programs. These use the effects of turbulence, buoyancy, warmth and resistance, and can be beneficial when recovering from surgery and/or injury. Even paralyzed limbs and muscles can benefit from this.

5) Hydrotherapy is often the treatment of choice when faced with the early post-surgical or "deconditioned" patient. The deconditioning process occurs "naturally" and rapidly when there is total inactivity for a period of time, or where the level of pain is high, resulting in the loss of muscle strength, joint flexibility and the loss of normal function. It is not uncommon for the patient to be unable to apply themselves in a traditional exercise program, either through pain, lack of strength or motivation.

Reiki Healing: Pronounced (ray-kee) is a gentle hands-on healing modality, which is delivered just inches above the body and can help restores spiritual equilibrium, and activates the body's own natural ability to heal itself. The name Reiki originates from the Japanese 'rei', meaning "universal" and 'ki', meaning "energy".

Reiki can be beneficial in reducing the pain of aching muscles, arthritis, toothaches, headaches (migraines), back pain and numbness from nerve damage. It can accelerate the healing of cuts, burns, broken bones, flu, nausea, allergies, and chronic illness like Fibromyalgia, Lupus and MS. Reiki has also been beneficial when treating such painful conditions as severe burns where touching the body could be excruciating, Reiki can be delivered just inches above the body.

"This is one treatment that I am yet to try, but would definitely like to explore this option further. Another one for the list of things to do!"

Basically, there is a whole host of different alternative therapies to try. By individually exploring these other options, you like my self may find a therapy that really helps you to cope with the fibromyalgia, which may make living with this condition easier. Below is a short description of a few of the various therapies available.

Bach Flower Remedies – First developed in the 1930s by Dr Edward Bach, the Bach flower remedies are based on the theory that there are seven major emotional groupings under which people could be classified. Using his knowledge of homoeopathy, Dr. Bach formulated a plant or flower based remedy to treat each of the emotional states. There are 38 different remedies, including:

Cherry Plum – Used for fear of the mind giving way

Gorse – Used for hopelessness and despair

Hornbeam – Used for procrastination, tiredness at the thought of doing something

Mimulus – Used for fear of known things

Mustard – Used for deep gloom for no reason

Oak – Used for the plodder who keeps going past the point of exhaustion

Olive – Used for exhaustion following mental or physical effort

Red Chestnut – Used for over concern for the welfare of loved ones

Sweet Chestnut – Used for extreme mental anguish, when everything has been tried
and there is no light left

Bio Energy – This is a complementary therapy based on ancient theory that all illness is caused by an imbalance of the body's energy flow, which can be caused by many problems including, anxiety. This therapy is implemented by the therapist discovering the energy flow circulating in and around the body using various hand movements using techniques based on the aura and charkas. Bio-Energy has been used for many ailments ranging from eczema to back problems.

Biofeedback Therapy – This is becoming more popular in the treatment of certain diseases and painful conditions, including fibromyalgia. Biofeedback uses techniques where the person learns to alter their own health by using the information from their own body signals.

Biomagnetic Therapy – Also referred to as magnetic field therapy and electromagnetic therapy has a history dating back thousands of years to Africa, where the 'Blood Stone' an ancient magnetic stone was discovered. Other ancient civilizations including the Chinese, Egyptians, Greeks, Hebrews, Indians and Tibetans have documented use of magnetism as part of their healing practices and lifestyles. Even Cleopatra is said to have worn one on her forehead as an anti-aging therapy.

Magnetic Therapy is used to relieve symptoms of many health conditions without medicines and works by reviving, reforming and promoting the body's growth of cells, rejuvenating tissues and increasing the number of healthy blood corpuscles and increases oxygen levels.

Chinese Herbal Medicine (RCHM) – This is a complete medical therapy that is capable of treating a very wide range of conditions including, chronic fatigue syndrome, depression, irritable bowel syndrome, osteoarthritis and rheumatoid arthritis. Treatments include herbal therapy, acupuncture, dietary therapy and exercises in breathing and movement (tai chi and qi gong).

Chinese herbal medicine is based on the concepts of 'Yin' and 'Yang' and is aimed to understand and treat the many ways in which the balance and harmony between the two may be undermined and the ways in which a person's 'Qi', or vitality may be affected.

Dance & Movement Therapy – People use movement to help meet their physical and emotional needs and if aligned with the mind's thoughts, then the body's natural expression will flow effortlessly. However, if an incongruity between the body and mind goes un-addressed it will inevitably lead to various internal conflicts, which can include emotional pain and discomfort, and in some cases the intra-psychic struggle can cause interpersonal problems, such as anxiety, depression, fear, physical pain, stress and in some cases, chronic disease.

Combining movement and traditional counselling techniques to address symptoms, such as those mentioned the above symptoms, through the use of dance and movement therapy, the individual can further their emotional, social, cognitive and physical integration and regain harmony in their lives.

"Remember, before trying any type of therapy or treatment, please remember to seek advice from your Doctor."

Emotional Freedom Technique (EFT) – This is one of the new discoveries in Meridian Therapies which can help with the effects of anger, depression, fears, phobias, trauma, stress and other emotional issues. This therapy is not perfect, but it has been known to work where everything else fails and can be used on psychological, physical and neuro-physiological problems.

This new approach covers all 14 meridian lines of the body using a tapping procedure. Think of it as a psychological version of acupuncture, except that needles aren't required. Instead, you 'tune in' to your emotional problem while stimulating the stress relief points by tapping on them with your fingertips. This provides a meridian 'balancing effect' that replaces emotional distress with a form of peace.

With this form of therapy:

1) The results can be long lasting.
2) The process is relatively gentle, and
3) Most people can apply the techniques to themselves, although for deeper problems the use of a skilled therapist is recommended.

The Emotional Freedom Technique can be used for problems such as:

Addictive Cravings

Anger

Anxiety & Panic Attacks

Depression & Sadness

Fear & Phobias

Grief & Loss

Insomnia

Stress and Trauma

This therapy is designed so that once you have learned the simple technique you can easily do it by yourself at home at anytime, and the techniques are comfortable, gentle, non-invasive and straight-forward to use.

Homoeopathy – Homoeopathy can often provide relief from the unpredictable, sometimes debilitating, aches and pains of fibromyalgia. However, it is recommended that you see a qualified homoeopath so that the correct treatment can be recommended and always consult with your doctor. Nutritional supplements, dietary monitoring, special types of exercise, and other natural approaches as already mentioned can also be beneficial and once consulted with your doctor, these may be used alongside other remedies.

Remedies I have tried with varying results include:

Arnica - Used when any body area feels bruised and sore, after exertion, overuse of muscles, or injury and for rheumatic joints with pain, heat and inflammation. On occasions *arnica* can be enough to soothe a chronic complaint, such as osteoarthritis.

Bryonia - This remedy is recommended for the sufferer who tries to remain as still as possible, especially if the slightest movement aggravates the pain. The person may feel extremely irritable and grumpy and unwilling to be touched. Warmth can often aggravate the problem, where as cool therapies may prove to be soothing. The sufferer may also find that pressure targeted on the painful areas, such as lying on them may help, because it minimizes any movement. May be beneficial for inflammation of the joint linings in arthritic and rheumatic conditions where symptoms include swelling, heat and pain.

Causticum – This remedy is used for soreness, weakness, and stiffness in the muscles, which tend to be worse from being cold and from overuse. Forearms may feel stiff, unsteady, and very weak, where as the leg muscles may feel sore and restless at night. Symptoms tend to be worse when the weather is dry and improve in wet weather, although getting wet can aggravate the pain and stiffness. Using warm therapies and making sure that the sufferer is warm in bed often relieve the discomfort.

Cimicifuga (also called Actae racemosa): People who need this remedy are often energetic and talkative, becoming depressed or fearful when physical problems trouble them. Soreness and stiffness of muscles may be accompanied by shooting pains and are usually aggravated by getting cold. The neck and spinal muscles can be very tight, and the person may have headaches and other problems during menstrual periods.

Rhus toxicodendron – This remedy is recommended if the sufferer feels very restless, with stiffness and soreness. They will find relief in warmth and by moving around. The symptoms can be aggravated by cold, damp weather and stiffness and/or pain are worse on waking in the morning, and after periods of rest. May be beneficial for conditions with symptoms of muscle and joint inflammation such as rheumatism, synovitis (inflammation of the synovial membranes surrounding the joints) and for osteoarthritis.

Ruta graveolens – This remedy may be beneficial for bone and joint injuries, disorders and those conditions affecting the ligaments, tendons and muscles where there is severe deep and tearing pain. May be helpful with fibromyalgia and is also used for synovitis and rheumatism.

Other homoeopathic remedies that may be beneficial include: **Kalmia latifolia,** used for rheumatic pains, **Ranunculus bulbosus,** used for rheumatism where symptoms include hot, tearing pain and **Rhododendron chrysanthemum,** which may be beneficial for rheumatism and arthritis where the main symptoms are hot swollen joints with severe pain.

Other therapies that may be benefical include:

Feng Shui

Meditation Therapy

Nutritional Therapy

Pain Management

Stress Management, and

Therapeutic Massage

Always consult with your medical practitioner before using any alternative therapy and only visit recommended and qualified therapists and healers. These suggestions should not be used to replace the treatment recommended by your doctor, but used as a complimentary therapy.

"Friends are angels who lift us to our feet when our wings have trouble remembering how to fly."

Crystal Healing

I decided to give crystal healing a small chapter of its own, as I am particularly interested in this form of alternative therapy and have found it to be personally beneficial in a rather soothing and gentle way.

What is Crystal Healing?

Crystal healing has been around for thousands of years and has been used as a holistic form of healing. It has been beneficial to the body's physical, emotional, mental and spiritual energies.

The human body is made up of vortexes of energy known as 'Chakras'. When a chakra becomes out of balance or blocked the body's natural flow of energy is disrupted causing symptoms such as pain, fatigue, listlessness, stress and depression.

Crystal healing works through vibration, as the crystals re-align the chakras located within the body, which then re-balance the bio-magnetic sheath that surrounds and inter-penetrates the body. During the healing process, the positive energy flows between the therapist and the person being treated.

Crystal healing is suitable for people of all ages and can assist with various types of health conditions. It can also be used as a general therapy to help re-charge the body and restore natural balance, harmony and wellbeing.

The beauty of this type of therapy is that it does not interfere with any conventional medication being taken. However, please note that healers are not qualified to diagnose health conditions, so your conventional doctor must still be top of your list. Remember, crystal healing is a complementary therapy which works alongside your conventional medicines.

My favourite crystals/stones are:

Amethyst: Try sleeping with a piece of amethyst under your pillow as it is beneficial for intuitive dreams and inspired thoughts. It is also known to soothe and calm the mind, raise your spirits, increase your level of intuitive awareness and protect from negative vibrations. This crystal is ideal for meditation. On a spiritual plane Amethyst is particularly useful for meditation.

Blue Lace Agate: This is a calming stone and is excellent for meditation and reducing the level of stress in the body. It may also be used to reduce infections, inflammations and fevers.

Crystal healing can be used for many different ailments, but like all therapies, whether alternative or conventional, the results and benefits experienced by every individual vary greatly. If using crystals then purchasing good quality stones and caring for them properly is important.

Hematite: This stone can bring about a calm mental state, improve memory, mental focus and concentration, support self-confidence and increase the effectiveness of logical processes of the brain and has a reputation for helping people bring order to mentally chaotic situations by drawing tension out of the body, neutralizing negativity and releasing any anger. Some believe it has the power to increase mental function and be able to improve memory, mathematical processes, logic, creativity and mental dexterity. Personally, I find it a beneficial aid in meditation and many healers recognize it for calming the mental state, tuning the consciousness and increasing the pathways that lead to inner knowledge.

The following crystals may be beneficial for Fibromyalgia:

Clear Quartz and Rose Quartz
Tiger eye
Morganite
Citrine
Hematite
Obsidian

Emerald
Sodalite
Amethyst
Amber
Laboradoite
Lapis Lazuli

For Arthritis:

Amethyst
Copper
Gold
Malachite
Black Tourmaline
Lapis Lazuli
Chrysocolla
Boji Stones
Green Calcite
Dolomite
Amber
Azurite
Petrified Wood

For Back Pain and/or Problems:

Fluorite
Lodestone
Obsidian
Calcite (especially orange or green)

For Chronic Fatigue:

Amethyst
Aquamarine
Rose Quartz
Orange Calcite
Aragonite
Ruby
Rhodochrosite
Boji stones

For Concentration:

Malachite
Flourite
Hematite

For Depression:

Kunzite
Citrine
Lepediolite
Rose quartz
Black Tourmaline
Peridot
Botswana Agate
Eliat Stone,Gold
Jet
Lapis Lazuli
Moonstone
Quartz
Platinum

To Boost Energy Levels:

Ruby
Rhodochrosite
Boji stones

For Meditation:

Amethyst
Yellow Calcite
Celestite
Azurite
Labradorite
Chrysocolla

Blue Tiger's Eye
Lapis Lazuli
Turquoise
Blue Fluorite
Quartz
Hawk's Eye
Apophyllite
Blue Sapphire
Selenite

For Memory:

Carnelian
Emerald
Onyx

For General Pain Relief:

Lapis Lazuli
Boji Stones
Green Calcite
Dolomite
Amber
Amethyst
Hematite
Howlite
Mugglestone

To get the most out of this type of therapy, I recommend that you see a therapist who is experienced in crystals and their healing properties. I have added two links to the resource page that provide a directory of various complementary therapists from around the world.

Conventional Treatments:

This is probably the shortest section of my book, as I personally try to avoid conventional drugs as often as possible for a more natural alternative, as already discussed. However, like everyone who suffers with fibromyalgia, the need for painkillers is necessary for those extremely bad days. And just lately that need has increased. More my fault for trying to do too much, so it's back to my old routine instead of trying to push myself that bit more.

Having tried a variation of over the counter and prescription medications, I was prescribed the prescription drug Co-Codamol 30/500mg, containing Paracetamol 500mg and Codeine Phosphate Hemihydrate 30mg in each tablet. On the bad days I would take the full daily recommendation of 8 tablets, although I did try to avoid this, as taking a high dosage of strong painkillers over a long period of time may lead to other health problems, such as damaging the stomach lining and aiding the development of stomach ulcers.

Whilst writing this book, I unfortunately needed to see my doctor again because the pain wasn't improving with the co-codamol alone. So at an appointment in September 2005, my doctor implemented all the usual examinations and prescribed another drug which could be taken along side the co-codamol for more effect. Dicloflex 50mg can be taken three times a day and contains the main ingredient of 'Diclofenac Sodium' and is used as a pain relief and inflammatory medicine for rheumatic diseases and musculoskeletal conditions such as, arthritis, lower back pain and dislocations, etc.

My doctor also requested that an up to date set of blood tests where taken, but they came back with normal results, which I didn't need a doctor to tell me that! So mixing the two prescribed medications still had no effect, and in fact made me feel twice as bad, as well as giving me severe stomach pains, headaches and nausea. So again I decided to come off the Dicloflex and stick to the co-codamol, because at least this drug doesn't increase my symptoms. January 2006, the pain increased further, so it was yet another visit to my local Doctor, where I requested to be referred to a new rheumatologist and where my journey of health continues. At the time of writing this section in my book I was waiting to receive an appointment to see a consultant. My Doctor gave a waiting time of up to 10 weeks. So at this stage I had decided that, if I didn't hear within this time period, then I would pay to see a rheumatologist privately.

Other conventional medications that I have tried over the years include:

Ibuprofen

Codeine

Paracetamol

Aspirin

Panadol

Buprenorphine Transdermal

Tramadol Hydrochloride and

Salazopyrin® EN (Sulphasalazine)*

I have also tried several ointments, but these tend to have very little effect.

These have included:

Ibugel

Deep Heat

Algesal

As mentioned in the previous chapter, when requiring the use creams or lotions, I use the natural ointment 'Emu Oil', which is warm and soothing to use.

In the battle to find a treatment that is suitable to the individual sufferer, doctors will prescribe various treatments over a period of time to see which provides the best response. These can range from:

Analgesics: Which are used to treat and/or prevent pain. However, they only work with some people.

Anti-inflammatory Medication: These tend to only provide partial pain relief to sufferers. This is because there are no signs of inflammation with the condition fibromyalgia.

Anti-depressants: These can be used to try and improve sleep patterns and lessen pain, and the doses recommended are significantly lower than the doses of medication taken by patients who actually suffer from depression. Personally, I found that they made no improvement on my own sleep disturbance and chose to again use more natural alternatives.

Please Note: That taking conventional sleeping tablets are not recommended as these can be habit-forming and like most medications when taken far too regularly, they can become non-effective.

Ironically, as already mentioned, with many conventional medications the possible side effects can be similar to the symptoms that fms sufferers experience, so finding a treatment to suit is a challenge in its self.

<u>**For example:**</u>

Co-Codamol has several possible side effects including:

Allergic Reaction including Itching
Confusion
Constipation
Dizziness

Dicloflex has side effects that mirror some of the symptoms seen with fibromyalgia, including, but not inclusive:

Anxiety
Confusion
Constipation
Depression
Dizziness
Fatigue
Headaches
Itching
Nausea
Sleeplessness
Trembling

Sulphasalazine which from the latter part of 2006 has been my most recent medication, taken alongside my painkillers can create the side effects:

Abdominal Pain
Diarrhoea
Dizziness
Headaches
Nausea, and
Rashes

However, it can also occasionally affect the blood count (which means fewer blood cells are produced). Conditions such as sore throats, infections, fevers and unexplained bruising needs to be reported to my rheumatology consultant, and because of the side effects of sulphasalazine on the blood and liver I need to have regular blood tests to monitor my condition and the effects of this particular drug.

If the Sulphasalazine fails to bring any relief, then my rheumatology consultant would like to give Methotrexate a try, but again this drug can affect the amount of blood cells produced. Taking conventional medication can be a battle to alleviate your diagnosed conditions with trying to prevent other conditions developing. It's just another vicious circle with these side-effects providing further health risks, so I do prefer the alternative treatment route where possible.

――――――――――――――――――

*** Chapter Footnote:** The Sulphasalazine was prescribed in November 2006 and is my latest medication, which is taken with these combined pain relief drugs, Tramadol Hydrochloride and Paracetamol. The Sulphasalazine is quite a new drug and can reduce the symptoms and slow the progress of rheumatoid arthritis and other forms of arthritis by helping to reduce the inflammation in joints and decreasing pain, swelling and stiffness. However, as with all drugs there can be side affects and I am being closely monitored by my Rheumatology consultant and GP.*

Fibromyalgia and Sex

Strangely sex is one of those topics that many people find uncomfortable to discuss, even to their nearest and dearest, and when you have a medical condition, this makes the process even more difficult to discuss and participate. Sex is also viewed differently by couples and its importance in a relationship varies from couple to couple. Some enjoy sex regularly, others less frequently such as monthly and there are couples who have a happy and fulfilling relationship without the sexual intimacy, being content to simply cuddle, hold hands and exchange kisses, without the desire to engage in full sexual intercourse. Which ever way you choose to enjoy each others company as a couple, discussing this subject is important to avoid confusion and psychological problems developing.

Fibromyalgia and Arthritis can at times interfere with the normal process of intimacy. However, with a little understanding, some thought and planning the natural relationship between two people can be experienced with little or no pain or discomfort from the person's medical symptoms. I'm not saying it is easy as the new way of thinking and participating is a learning process to both people and many couples do naturally find it difficult until they have mastered the changes *(11)*. However, looking at the positive side of building on your relationship, so that both people can be sexually satisfied is that exploring new techniques can also be enjoyable, but to achieve this you do need to learn to communicate with each other, so that you both understand how the other is feeling emotionally and physically.

Two of the main difficulties that sufferers experience are fatigue and pain, which affects our sexuality and unfortunately some medications taken to help Fibromyalgia and Arthritis, can also affect the natural desire for intimacy. This combined with the pain experienced, can therefore lead the person suffering with these conditions into not wishing to participate sexually. Naturally by avoiding communication with your partner, they can begin to feel angry, frustrated and rejected which can then lead to problems within the relationship.

For the partner of the person suffering with these conditions, learning to accept that they may not be in the mood or that they are having a bad day with their condition is an important fact of life to remember.

Many problems related to sexual intimacy can develop with Fibromyalgia and Arthritis and pain is one of the main problems, as the sufferer can experience symptoms such as, muscles which can painfully ache during intimacy from the pressure, especially around the lower back and pelvic muscles, and this can lead to painful intercourse. Another symptom is muscle cramp during intercourse which can also create problems (*12*).

The second main problem is fatigue, as most sexual activity requires a large amount of energy, and this alone can be a problem for people suffering from Fibromyalgia and/or Arthritis, as they will without doubt suffer with fatigue due to their disturbed sleep patterns. Again some medications used to treat these conditions can also interfere with sexual responsiveness, such as those used to increase the body's serotonin level (*13*). Women may lack sexual desire (libido), or may be unable to achieve an orgasm. Male sufferers of these conditions may lack libido, or have difficulty achieving erections, and the side effects from some medications can also cause extreme sedation, preventing your partner from being sexually alert.

Emotional problems may also be present, such as depression, negative self–image, anxiety or fear of rejection, and even though your partner may be able to physically respond sexually, the following points must be considered.

1) Self–perception
2) Increased vulnerability and,
3) Emotional pain can all limit the interest in intimacy.

Then to add even more problems, some treatments prescribed for depression can also create further problems in the relationship, as some anti-depressant medications can decrease sexual desire and function.

Finally, the daily problems associated with Fibromyalgia and Arthritis combined with the fear of causing your partner any physical pain may further decrease the natural course of intimacy and sexual contact (*14*).

Here are some tips that may help:

1) You should both learn more about the sufferers condition, so that you can discuss and plan an alternative approach which may enable you both to enjoy a more fulfilling sexual relationship.

2) Be prepared to accept the emotional changes, such as anger, blame, depression and frustration. These feelings of resentment need to be discussed and worked on if any improvement is to be achieved. Avoiding this can cause serious problems in your relationship. This is something that both people will need to understand as it will at some stage affect both the individuals.

3) Both people need to look after their health and looks, as this can help to improve their self-image and regular exercise is important, especially for the person with the fibromaylgia or arthritis. The other positive side to this tip is that exercising together can be a shared opportunity and enjoyable, that may bring you closer together as a couple.

4) Remember to communicate with each other, as this is one of the most important facts in satisfying any sexual relationship (*15*). Encourage new ideas about things you and your partner would like to try, to compensate for the changes the fibromyalgia and/or arthritis has made in your sexuality. Most of all "Consider this an adventure well worth your time and energy" (*16*).

5) Remember to be creative and plan ahead. It's no good if the sufferer is physically exhausted or having a bad day of pain. Choose a time when you are both in the right frame of mind for intimacy and be imaginative in setting the right mood, with scented candles, soothing music, taking a warm bath, etc. The room should be set at a comfortable temperature and away from any drafts. Experiment with pillows and other soft furnishings to support the body and create a comfortable setting.

6) Remember that certain positions may be painful for the person with fibromyalgia or arthritis, so finding comfortable positions will mean taking time to experiment to see what positions are more suitable. "Positions that involve arching the back, straightening the legs, twisting the spine, or positions that require a lot of support from only one leg or one arm can be often painful for an individual with these conditions and can lead to muscle cramps" (*17*). Instead, experiment with side–lying positions, lying on the back with knees bent, sitting positions, standing positions, or positions where the back is supported. Avoid staying in one position too long, as this again can lead to muscle cramps. Learn to talk openly with your partner and discuss what postitions hurt. "Remember that sexual activity will not damage fibromyalgia muscles so have fun" (*18*).

7) Another point to consider is that intercourse isn't the only way to be intimate with one another. So try having some fun by exploring new ways of pleasuring each other. This can range from a gentle massage, cuddling, kissing to sharing a hot tub. Remember, penetrative sex is not the only way to achieve and enjoy sexual fulfillment. Mutual masturbation is rewarding and may be particularly appropriate where vaginal sex is difficult and/or uncomfortable. I am sure that you can think of others if you let your imagination flow. However, communication with your partner is just so important when changing the way you approach your sexual activities, so don't forget to reassure your partner that you love and trust them. If you are uncomfortable, tell your partner and suggest other alternatives you are willing to try.

8) Finally, if you are both concerned that fibromyalgia, arthritis and/ or depression may be affecting your sex life, don't be embarrassed to seek professional advice as this is a perfectly normal approach to the problem. Your doctor can provide you with information and can alter medications and dosages, which may alleviate any negative side effects and sex therapy counselors may be able to help you both communicate with one another, and provide new ideas for intimacy. Fibromyalgia and arthritis support groups can also provide an opportunity for couples to meet others with similar experiences. Your local health clinic will be able to provide you with contacts for counselors and support groups in your community.

Many books have also been published covering the subject of sexual intimacy and are widely available at libraries and bookstores, and the internet is another resource where you can get information about intimacy issues. For example, the Arthritis Foundation website has information about intimacy for arthritis and fibromylagia sufferers, and the Arthritis Research Campaign publish a very good booklet called "Sexuality and Arthritis".

"Achieving can only begin with Believing"

My Fibro A-Z

This is my own personal Fibro A-Z guide. However, please note that I make no claim that any of the remedies or points mentioned will help with your own fibromyalgia. They are simply there for information. However, they are worth considering with the approval of your Doctor, as I have found some of them to be very beneficial*.

~

Anti-inflammatory Medication - Many doctors disagree that fibromyalgia creates inflammation, but I personally disagree with this as feels my muscles, tendons and bones often feel inflamed! However, some recent reports indicate that fibromyalgia may be an inflammatory condition caused by 'Mycoplasmas'. These are mutated bacteria and viruses that invade certain glands of the brain and even organs of the body. So I use a ***Natural Anti-inflammatory** that I believe can be helpful and there are many you can try including Devils Claw and Glucosamine. People with fibromyalgia can also suffer from other inflammatory conditions such as arthritis and tendonitis.

*Antioxidants – These are nutrients obtained from our food and drink. They help reduce cell damage from harmful toxins and help prevent oxidation by neutralizing free radicals which can react with and damage other body substances. Common antioxidants include Beta-carotene, Ginkgo Biloba, Grape Seed Extract, Lutein, Selenium and the Vitamins A, C and E.

*Be Happy – Having fibromyalgia is 'not' a 'mind-over-matter' condition and those people that have never experienced fms cannot even start to understand what we sufferers go through on a daily basis. However, I am a strong believer that keeping happy is one of life's great healers, so for heaven sake cheer yourself up and watch a funny movie, or read a comical or inspirational book. Look back and think of all those funny and happy memories, sing and laugh. "A giggle a day may help to keep the Doctor away!" A positive outlook on life, being happy and enjoying some humour certainly helps me get through the worst periods of pain and discomfort.

*Books – There are many books available on fibromyalgia that have been written by medical doctors regarding conventional and alternative treatments. It's nice to see that some ideas which have helped me and others with this condition are actually being published by professionals in the health sector. I have placed a list of my recommended books further on in this publication.

However, one recent book I purchased deserves an extra mention. *Effortless Pain Relief – By Dr Ingrid Bacci, Bantam 2005,* is certainly worth purchasing. This book is based on the principle that when we understand the causes of pain, we open the door to developing effective techniques for managing and even eliminating pain from our lives. Whilst exploring the concept of how stress and an unhealthy lifestyle can contribute to sometimes chronic conditions, this inspired guide also offers techniques and advice on how to alleviate specific problems such as arthritis, fibromyalgia and back pain.

Boswellin – This is an aromatic herb which has anti-inflammatory and analgesic properties. Many people find it beneficial for stiff joints and it is used for conditions such as Rheumatoid Arthritis and Osteoarthritis.

*Chondroitin Sulphate – This is a major substance of the connective tissues, which make up the body's joints. Taking this as a supplement can help to promote tissue repair and healing, whilst improving the condition of the connective tissues. This is often taken combined with the supplement Glucosamine.

Cold Compress – Gel compress packs can be stored in the fridge or freezer and applied to the back of the neck when you're lying down. Cold gel packs help to slow down your own thoughts, providing a calmer more relaxed mood. You may find it helps you to drop off to sleep. However, a word of warning - If you keep your gel pack in the freezer, wrap a cloth over it to avoid damaging delicate skin or blood vessels from the intense cold.

Doctors – Sadly, some doctors still seem uninformed on how to treat fibromyalgia and with the mixed symptoms, many seem to opt for the first choice of prescribing muscle relaxants, anti-depressants, anti-inflammatories, sleeping tablets and pain relief medication, of which many prove unhelpful and most have alarming side effects that can be not only unpleasant, but can carry risks attached to them. Unfortunately, there are a number of people with fibromyalgia that don't get better and continue to return to their doctors with various health problems, which are not helped by a few doctors who still have a tendency to blame the FMS sufferer, rather than admit that they don't know how else to treat the condition. There are even reports of some fibromyalgia sufferers being told that, *"It's all in your mind,"* or *"I'm afraid you will have to learn to live with it!"* So if you are not happy with the help you are getting from your doctor, find another more understanding medical practitioner who is up to date with all the latest treatments.

Depression – This can be a problem for many FMS sufferers, and is caused by a disturbance in brain chemicals brought on by the continuing lack of restorative sleep, and we all know that without this our body's simply can not function properly. Other reasons for the onset of depression can include, feeling a sense of loss. This in itself can be overwhelming and plays host to not only our health, but to our lifestyles, our ability to think clearly, our careers and in many cases even our spouses, friends or family members who simply fail to understand fully on how you feel. Finding that little miracle to help you get the restorative sleep needed is a tough battle.

Sleeping tablets can be addictive if used too often, anti-depressants can also have some worrying side, including anxiety, depression, drowsiness, restlessness and even the inability to sleep, which simply defeats the object of taking them. Personally, the anti-depressants never worked for me, all they seem to do was make me feel worse than I did anyway. Finding a natural alternative to help you sleep and medical support from your doctor is important. If you do get depressed, again you should seek help before you sink to deep. Once at rock bottom, it's hard to pick yourself up.

*Devils Claw – This is a traditional herbal remedy, which is popular for treating Arthritis and Rheumatic Pain. This remedy helps to promote joint, tendon and ligament health and is a natural anti-inflammatory. This is one of my favourite natural health remedies that I use often. Even my dogs take this supplement for their arthritic conditions and their mobility has improved greatly to the extent that their veterinary prescribed medication has now been reduced. It is certainly worth a try.

*Drink Water – This may seem obvious, but not enough people drink enough pure water. This is important, as water naturally helps to flush all those unwanted toxins out of the body. If you dislike the taste of ordinary tap water, then there are plenty of bottled varieties on the market to choose from.

Echinacea – Another herbal remedy that has anti-viral, anti-bacterial and anti-fungal properties. Can be used at times of physical and emotional stress as a 'pick-me-up' and apparently can be used to treat the condition Candida (yeast infection).

*Exercise – A little is better than nothing, as long as you don't push your self too far and to the point of increasing your pain and discomfort. The longer you sit idle, the stiffer you will become and the pain will increase. Take a short walk and attempt some gentle stretching exercises, remembering to use warming up and cooling down exercises so as not to injure your self further. Try gentle yoga, tai-chi or even water aerobics.

On the other hand, try to avoid any activity that is repetitive, such as typing, cross stitch, embroidery, etc… If you do find that some of your activities are repetitive, then make sure you stop regularly, implement some gentle stretching exercises and get up and move around so you don't become stiff, which can lead to pain and discomfort. If you work in an office, encourage your office colleagues to join in with the stretching exercises, they too will feel more relaxed, refreshed, less stiff and hopefully a little more positive with their working thoughts.

*Essential Oils - Try therapeutic grade essential oils, as some people with fms have found these to be beneficial. I personally use Lavender and Helichrysum to help with my insomnia, to relax and as a natural anti-inflammatory which can help with the pain and discomfort. Remember, oils should always be combined with either massage lotion or almond oil, when using them directly on your body.

*Feverfew – An ancient herbal remedy with anti-inflammatory properties. I find this a great headache remedy, even for those real thumper headaches, such as migraines and apparently it is also a beneficial treatment for arthritis.

*Fibro Friends – Making friends with other sufferers can help you feel less isolated, as they will understand how you feel and will be sensitive to the pain you feel. Many through their own experiences will have lots of helpful tips to help you cope with your own symptoms. There are many places you can make new fibro friends, including forums and local support groups.

*Glucosamine – This is now available as tablets in a vegetarian version. Glucosamine helps to maintain the 'Connective Tissues' and 'Joints', which are continuously regenerating. You can purchase this supplement with the added anti-oxidant 'Vitamin C', or as I do take it separately. These supplements can also be combined with 'Chondroitin', which is a constituent of the connective body tissues. You can even buy Glucosamine Joint Patches which may help to relieve muscular tension and discomfort around the ankles, elbows, wrists, knees, neck, shoulders and back. I have used these, but the effect on the discomfort varies on how bad a day I am having, but still worth a try. These products are available from most reputable health food stores, but do shop around as the prices can vary considerably.

*Heat Treatment – Taking a warm or hot bath can sometimes relieve the stiffness and discomfort of fibromyalgia for short periods. Alternatively, try a heat pack which can be beneficial, especially on cold days. I use a 'Hot-Pak' 100% natural herbal heat pack which contains a blend of wheat grains and a selection of relaxing herbs, including Lavender. Heat packs can be beneficial in many common ailments including, arthritis, rheumatism, migraine, menstrual pain, stress and tension. This particular make can also be used as an ice pack by freezing it inside another bag for 3 hours. This can be beneficial for ailments such as, bruising, sprains and swellings. I simply add a few drops of lavender oil to refresh the fragrance as required, which also has the benefit of helping me relax of a night. (www.hot-pak.com)

*5-Hydroxytryptophan (5HTP) – Is a natural mood enhancer used to alleviate the symptoms of depression, reduces the sensation of pain and promotes sleep. This substance naturally occurs in the body, where it is converted into the neurotransmitter, Serotonin.

Iron - Avoid nutritional supplements containing iron, unless you have had a blood test that shows you are anemic and it has been recommended by your doctor. Be aware of Hemochromotosis which is a health condition caused by excessive iron in the body, which has similar symptoms to those associated with fibromyalgia.

Joint Mobility – Naturally as we get older our body's age, resulting in a decrease in the production and maintenance of the connective tissues such as the muscles and cartilage. Taking supplements can help, and these include Boswellin, Celery, Chondroitin Sulphate, Cod Liver Oil, Copper, Glucosamine, MSN and Omega 3 Fatty Acids.

Knees – This may seem like common sense, but it so easy to simply kneel down. You should avoid kneeling where possible and if you do need to go down into this position, kneel on a good supportive cushion. This will help to protect your knees, absorb the pressure and lessen the discomfort. If at night when you are trying to sleep and you find that lying on your side increases the discomfort around your knees, simply add a soft cushion or pillow between the knees to disperse the pressure and weight of the top leg. This really does help, especially if you find sleeping on your back a problem.

*Lecithin – This is a lipid which is essential to every single body cell. This supplement may help to increase energy levels, boost the immune system and relieve the symptoms associated with Chronic Fatigue Syndrome. It has also been known to improve short-term memory and endurance.

*Low Fat Diet - Exercise can cause pain and discomfort, and because of this a lot of people with fibromyalgia become inactive, which leads to increases in weight. Try eating regular, well-balanced meals that are low in fat and sugar to help keep your blood sugar levels stable. This will help you maintain a healthy body weight. Remember, toxins are stored in fat cells, so it is common sense not to become overweight.

*Mental Relaxation - Allow your mind to unwind in the evening, by listening to gentle, relaxing music, as this will help you to fall asleep. Always avoid anything that is mentally stimulating, such as rushing around, studying or catching up with business paperwork.

Massage – This is one therapy that you can involve your spouse or other family member. If you prefer, you can also enjoy a massage from a qualified therapist. This is a good option, as most therapists will understand where the fibro trigger points are and will use a good technique to help alleviate the pain.

MSM - Methylsulfonylmethane is a naturally occurring rich sulphur substance found in all plants and animals. It is known to boost collagen production and may be beneficial to people suffering with connective tissue disorders and arthritis.

Noise – Many fibro sufferers are sensitive to noise and/or may suffer from the condition tinnitus (ringing in the ears). So try to avoid places where there will be loud bangs or a lot of noise disturbance. However, here in rural Lincolnshire, finding complete peace can be a problem with the military and their low flying jets frequently passing over the roof of your home… At night when you are trying to drop off to sleep, try wearing soft foam ear plugs, which are available from your pharmacist.

*Nutritional Supplements -- These are based on individual requirements, as we are all different. However, some fibro sufferers have found them to be beneficial. Other supplements that I use regularly include, Evening Primrose Oil, Collagen and Vitamin B.

*Omega 3, 6 and 9 – These are EFA's or essential fatty acids which are derived from nuts, seeds and some types of fish. Our body's are unable to produce these alone, although our body's need them for cell regeneration and health. They have anti-inflammatory properties and have been found to be beneficial in relieving digestive upsets, arthritis and depression.

*Pain Relieving Gels – Worth trying, as these can help to relieve a lot of aches and pains associated with FMS, as well as from overworked muscles, strains, etc. For a natural alternative, try emu oil which has anti-inflammatory properties and contains linolenic acid which is known to ease muscle and joint pain.

*Posture - Many people with fibromyalgia have poor posture due to the increase of muscle strength and effort it takes to hold their body's erect. Learn to sit up, or stand up straight as having good posture is important in reducing further problems associated with the neck and back.

*Probiotics – These are 'good' bacteria derived from some bifidobacteria and microflora lactobacilli and are found in many foods, such as yoghurts. Research has shown that probiotics can help to alleviate the symptoms associated with IBS (Irritable Bowel Syndrome), which is a condition many fibro sufferers have. One of my favourite yoghurts is Yeo Valley Organic Fat Free Bio Live in vanilla flavour and it's delicious with some fresh fruit. This yoghurt contains the live cultures, Lactobacillus, Acidophilus and Bifidobacterium. One other good point is that it is gluten free. (www.yeo-organic.co.uk)

Quality of Life – Don't get n a rut. Always think positive even on those bad days when the pain is especially bad. Keep smiling, set yourself targets and get out and do a bit of exercise. Staying in doors vegetating will only make you experience more stiffness and the pain more unbearable.

*Reduce Stress - Many fibromyalgia sufferers are people who aim high to achieve what they want and have a high level of energy, and because of this we can be prone to simply doing too much, which can encourage high stress levels. Learn to say 'No' and allow yourself daily space to relax, laugh and simply to be you. If possible, cut your working hours, go self-employed or stop working altogether, so that you can have time to manage your fibromyalgia.

Relax – Learn to relax by allowing yourself some personal time to lie down and rest. This doesn't mean you have to sleep, as most doctors prefer you not to sleep during the day as it conflicts with their programme to get you back into a normal sleep pattern. However, this failed for me, so I prefer to get some sleep when I can and if that means having a sleep during the day, then that is just what I do and feel better for it. Learn to relax by gently slowing down your mind, by pushing hectic and negative thoughts to one side and thinking of more peaceful thoughts that bring calm and help to release all that built up tension.

Many FMS sufferers, including myself need these short periods of rest to get through the day. If you can't lie down, then sit in a comfortable chair, or lay your head down on your desk and switch off your phone to avoid being disturbed. There is nothing strange in this, as many people, including those non-sufferers take naps every day to restore their mental faculties and energy levels. Just take a look on the train and see how many business people have their eyes closed.

Research – Thankfully, more and more research is taking place on this condition. Fibromyalgia is a condition built around many points, including auto-immune, hormones and neurological areas. The more you research your condition, the more information you will have to help you cope and manage your condition. Don't just rely on the help of your doctor. It's up to you to educate your self on fibromyalgia, allowing you to work knowledgeably alongside any medical support.

Sleep - Tackling insomnia will help to improve the symptoms associated with fibromyalgia. Consult with your doctor with regards to trying either melatonin or 5HTP which aid restorative sleep at night with no side effects the next day. I tried antidepressants for sleep, but quite frankly they made me feel worse than I felt before taking them, so I chose to try the more natural approach of 5HTP. However, please do note that most natural remedies are there simply as a support aid for sleep and may take several days to start working properly. One thing they will not do is knock you out like a sedative, but they can help you to feel more refreshed when you wake up, indicating that you have at least had some restorative sleep.

*Shoes - Be sensible and wear comfortable shoes with good support. High heels and platforms really do add stress to your muscles and tendons. Completely flat shoes can be as bad, so help your self by wearing the sort of shoes that fit the natural contour of your feet and don't induce pain and added stress to your feet and legs.

Smoking - Avoid it like the plague. How can anyone say they are serious about their health if they smoke, and that includes people with fibromyalgia? Smokers breathe in a vast amount of unhealthy free radicals with every single puff inhaled, and these free radicals greatly damage blood, tissues and cells.

Remember, smoking is a major factor in causing lung cancer, chronic bronchitis, emphysema, high blood pressure and strokes to name a few conditions.
Get motivated – Give Up the Cigarettes…

*Substance P - There may be abnormally low levels of blood flow in the parts of the brain that deal with pain in people with FMS! They may also have twice the level of a brain chemical called Substance P, which helps nervous system cells communicate with each other about painful stimuli. Elevated P levels may also produce the higher levels of pain throughout the body.

*Temperature – Make sure that when you do go to bed, your bedroom is neither, too hot or too cold as this will disturb sleep. An ideal temperature is 65-70°F.

T.E.N.S - Transcutaneous Electrical Nerve Stimulation is a recommended aid to pain relief. It works by eliminating the pain by transmitting tiny electrical messages to the nerve endings. This produces 'Endorphins' which are the body's natural pain killers and provides a soothing relief from various types of pain including, back pain, rheumatic, joint and muscle pain. This is something I hope to try.

Understanding – Gaining the support and understanding of family and friends is important in helping the sufferer cope with this painful condition. If you can't explain it to them, then send them a copy of the "Letter to the Normal" by Ronald J. Waller, located in the next chapter of this book.

*Valerian – This is another traditional herbal remedy which has been used for centuries to promote restful sleep. It is known to have powerful sedative properties, which can leave the person feeling refreshed and without the usual side effects of prescription or over the counter medications. This is something I have used regularly in the past and still do on occasions.

* Vinegar – Apple Cider Vinegar may bring some relief to pain. Mix 2 teaspoons of apple cider vinegar with 2 teaspoons of honey and dissolve in a small glass of warm water and drink twice a day. Hot vinegar may also help to bring pain relief by rubbing it into aching joints (*19*).

*Worry Time – We all know that if you have something on your mind, it can disturb your sleep. Allowing yourself 'worry time' during the day will help to prevent your mind wandering at night. Have a note pad and pen to hand and anything that comes into your mind right it down, so you can go back to it at your chosen 'worry time' and tackle the issue, whatever it may be.

X-rays & Scans – These will not diagnose fibromyagia. However, they are certainly worth having to rule out any other conditions, or forms of arthritis such as rheumatoid.

Yeast – An overgrowth of yeast **(candida albicans)** can cause similar symptoms to fibromyalgia and CFIDS! These include muscle and joint pain, difficulty concentrating, chronic fatigue, neurological disorders, insomnia, bowel dysfunction and a weakened immune system to name a few. If you crave sugar or carbohydrates, or have been taking antibiotics, you may have a yeast problem. You can try eliminating all sugar, fruit, honey, fructose, and fruit juice from your diet for a while to see if it helps your symptoms. Yeasts feed on sugar! You may feel worse before you feel better, however. Try some of the various probiotic foods, which contain beneficial microflora that can help control the yeast overgrowth (candidiasis).

*Zinc** – This is a naturally occurring mineral found in the body. It plays a vital role in the production, storage and secretion of hormones and aids cell replication, tissue repair and growth. Good zinc levels are essential to maintain all round health.

*ZNatural** *(The Original Patented Product)* & **Zeolite Liquid** – These are a group of minerals used for detoxifying the human body and may help to remove heavy metals, toxins and other compounds from the body, whilst supporting a healthy immune system and working as a powerful antioxidant. They work by attracting and buffering excess protons, which cause acidity and therefore may help with conditions such as, arthritis. I certainly feel a lot better since taking this product, as well as having more energy. The other reason for using this product, is that since losing my father to cancer, I want to try anything that may be a preventative measure for myself and more information on how zeolites can help can be found on the website 'Say No To Cancer' which is located in the resource section in this book.

A Letter to the Normal:

Making those people around you aware of how this condition affects you is not easy. However, sufferers around the world, my self included, do understand how difficult a task this is. I even find it hard explaining my symptoms to the doctor as at times there seems so many, or you wait for an appointment and when you get there you happen to be having a good day where the pain is less noticeable making you feel guilty for seeking help. If you are one of those people who find it hard to explain how you feel to family, friends and other non-sufferers that are associated with your daily life and to those people that do not really understand the effects of having fibromyalgia, then this letter may help to educate them. It's quite long, but well worth it and it really explains how fibro sufferers feel. However, please note that the following letter is copyrighted, but permission is granted to anyone who wishes to use it *(20).*

~ ~ ~

Hello Family, Friends, and Anyone Wishing to Know Me,

Allow me to begin by thanking you for taking the time out of your day to spend some time with me and get to know me better. A person's time is their most valuable asset and yours is appreciated.

I want to talk to you about Fibromyalgia (FM) and Chronic Myofascial Pain Syndrome (MPS). Many have never heard of these conditions and for those who have, many are misinformed. And because of this judgments are made that may not be correct... So I ask you to keep an open mind as I try to explain who I am and how FM/MPS has assaulted not only my life but those whom I love as well.

You see, I suffer from a disease that you cannot see; a disease that there is no cure for and that keeps the medical community baffled at how to treat and battle this demon, who's attacks are relentless. My pain works silently, stealing my joy and replacing it with tears. On the outside we look alike you and I; you wont see my scars as you would a person who, say, had suffered a car accident. You won't see my pain in the way you would a person undergoing chemo for cancer; however, my pain is just as real and just as debilitating. And in many ways my pain may be more destructive because people can't see it and do not understand....

Please don't get angry at my seemingly lack of interest in doing things; I punish myself enough I assure you. My tears are shed many times when no one is around. My embarrassment is covered by a joke or laughter, but inside I want to die....

Most of my "friends" are gone; even members of my own family have abandoned me. I have been accused of "playing games" for another's sympathy. I have been called unreliable because I am forced to cancel plans I made at the last minute because the burning and pain in my legs or arms is so intense I cannot put my clothes on and I am left in my tears as I miss out on yet another activity I used to love and once participated in with enthusiasm.

I feel like a child at times... Just the other day I put the sour cream I bought at the store in the pantry, on the shelf, instead of in the refrigerator; by the time I noticed it, it had spoiled. When I talk to people, many times I lose my train of thought in mid sentence or forget the simplest word needed to explain or describe something. Please try to understand how it feels to have another go behind me in my home to make sure the stove is off after I cook an occasional meal. Please try to understand how it feels to "lose" the laundry, only to find it in the stove instead of the dryer. As I try to maintain my dignity the Demon assaults me at every turn. Please try to understand....

Sleep, when I do get some, is restless and I wake often because of the pain the sheets have on my legs or because I twitch uncontrollably. I walk through many of my days in a daze with the Fibro-fog laughing at me as I stumble and grasp for clarity.

And just because I can do a thing one day, that doesn't mean I will be able to do the same thing the next day or next week. I may be able to take that walk after dinner on a warm July evening; the next day or even the in the next hour I may not be able to walk to the fridge to get a cold drink because my muscles have begun to cramp and lock up or spasm uncontrollably. And there are those who say "but you did that yesterday!" "What is your problem today?" The hurt I experience at those words scars me so deeply that I have let my family down again; and still they don't understand....

On a brighter side I want you to know that I still have my sense of humor. If you take the time to spend with me you will see that. I love to tell that joke to make another's face light up and smile at my wit. I love my kids and grandbabies and shine when they give me my hugs or ask me to fix their favorite toy. I am fun to be with if you will spend the time with me on my own playing field; is this too much to ask? I love you and want nothing more than to be a part of your life. And I have found that I can be a strong friend in many ways. Do you have a dream? I am your friend, your supporter and many times I will be the one to do the research for your latest project; many times I will be your biggest fan and the world will know how proud I am at your accomplishments and how honored I am to have you in my life.

So you see, you and I are not that much different. I too have hopes, dreams, goals... and this demon.... Do you have an unseen demon that assaults you and no one else can see? Have you had to fight a fight that crushes you and brings you to your knees? I will be by your side, win or lose, I promise you that; I will be there in ways that I can. I will give all I can as I can, I promise you that. But I have to do this thing my way. Please understand that I am in such a fight myself and I know that I have little hope of a cure or effective treatments, at least right now. Please understand....

Thank you for spending your time with me today. I hope we can work through this thing, you and I. Please understand that I am just like you... Please understand....

Copyright of www.fibrohugs.com -Written by Ronald J. Waller

"Friends are the flowers in life's garden"

Fibro Messages:

Since I first started out on the internet with my website *'Living with Fibromyalgia'* in 2004, which has now been updated and renamed to *'Fibromyalgia & Arthritis'* (www.fibromyalgiaandarthritis. co.uk), I have had many people contact me, either requiring advice for themselves or for someone they know who suffers with these conditions. I will always offer support where I can, as having a person who understands these conditions can be a great help, even if it just stops the other person from feeling so isolated. I hope that later this year the website forum will become more active, allowing sufferers, friends and family to leave messages and in doing so helping others who may venture down this journey of life in the battle of having FMS.

Here are just a few of the messages I receive each week. Naturally for confidentiality I have only used the person's name or internet alias and only part of my replies have been printed.

Email & Forum 2004:

"Hi A.J.

Came across your site today and believe that because of your understanding your may be able to advise. I have also sent an email to you with regards to this, but thought that my question and your reply may help others in my situation on the forum. I hope a question like this is ok to ask! But I am getting so depressed and annoyed with myself. I was diagnosed with FMS 8 months ago and am finding it increasingly difficult to have a normal relationship with my wife. Naturally we are both getting frustrated because I am either too tired and in too much discomfort or I simply cannot perform. Can you please explain why this is? Sorry to ask such a question to a lady but I find it hard to talk to people direct and at least you cannot see me or my embarrassment and no one knows who I am.

Thanks in advance".
Matrix (UK)

Reply:

You are more than welcome to ask these questions.

This is a perfectly normal reaction from both yourself and your wife, and something many FMS sufferers and their partners can associate with. You both really do need to sit down and discuss your emotions so that frustration can be released and allow you both too understand how the other is feeling. Your wife needs to understand that this is not your fault and needs to support and work with you on this.

Are you on any medication for this condition? If so here is some information that will help you understand why you cannot perform as well as before, and advice on what you should do next.

Medications known to cause Sexual Dysfunction:

Antidepressants: Most of the antidepressants do cause some sexual dysfunction to some degree. Some of the various antidepressants can cause premature-ejaculation and other problems. Effexor, Zoloft, and Paxil are the three highest in this category. Luvox, Prozac, and Celexa were next in line. Remeron and Wellbutrin show no complications with premature ejaculation. This is from a study by Dr. Caroline Dott & Dr. Andrew Dott *(21)*. Serezone caused no problems with ejaculation.

Some other sexual side effects which cause almost no desire, Zoloft, Effexor, rank the highest in this area. Prozac, Celexa, Wellbutrin, and Paxil are midrange. While Luvox and Serazone appeared to be the very least, to cause a lack of desire.

Paxil and Effexor were at the top reporting impotence Prozac, Celexa, Wellbutrin was midrange. Serezone and Luvox showed the least reporting of impotence.

However, this was just a study. Every medication will react differently in different people. Finding something that helps with your depression is very important in your treatment for fibromyalgia. Yet, when and if the pain subsides, and the time is right, you don't want a failure in the natural sexual pleasures between yourself and your wife. Do some research, dig around, and you will most likely have to try various antidepressants.

Pain Medication:

Pain medication can also affect your sex life. However, it is unique in the sense, some people it gives them impotence, and others it increases the sexual drives. One would think that just getting rid of the pain for a few hours, would be OK, but it is not. This another one of those things we all hear, you will have to find out what works for you, and discuss it with your doctor.

Feelings:

We've lost our power, our strength, our desire, our ability to love and be loved. Since some of our medications take away from our sexual lives, we often feel useless. No other word can describe it better. There is sometimes a never-ending fear looming over our heads, wondering if our spouses/partners will leave us, simply because we no longer function the way we used to, and this is a very natural emotion. Those who are single, often just give up on dating, because the "day" will come up, when the topic of sex is going to come up, and how do we handle that situation?

All these emotions stack up and the mere pressure of these feelings, let alone the side effects of medication are enough to cause a psychological dysfunction. They increase the stress, the medications decrease the ability for sexual relief, and where does that leave us? In the dark!

Sadly, there is unfortunately no quick answer to this dilemma.

Counseling will help, finding a local support group who will help, and working with your doctor to find the right combination that works, and decreases the over all side effects, will help also. Your doctor must be aware of what is going on with you, and therefore it is up to you to tell your doctor about these problems you are experiencing.

Email & Forum 2004:

"Thank you so much A.J for your detailed reply.

My wife and I sat and read it with interest and as you suggested have talked about our feelings which got everything into the open. I am on anti-depressants to try and help my sleep patterns and wasn't told about the side effects. We will be making a appointment with my GP so that we can discuss this and hopefully he will be able to give me something that will be less likely to affect my performance and also tell us of a local support group. Naturally now we have found your forum we will drop in often. I feel a lot happier today.

Thank you again for your kind and prompt answer and for understanding."

Matrix (UK)

Letter 2005:

"Having been diagnosed recently with FMS I was struggling to find sources of information until I came across your website. It's so comforting to know that you are not alone in the world with this condition and that there is always a fibro friend to listen and help you through the day. I just wanted to say thanks for giving me the inspiration to do something about my fibromyalgia, instead of sitting around hoping that it would go away."

Amy (UK)

Reply:

I am very pleased that my website has been informative and helpful to you, as well as encouraging you to motivate yourself instead of moping around, which would have made your symptoms worse over time, as a little gentle exercise will help to keep you mobile. You certainly are not alone and there are many people out there willing to help and provide friendly support.

Email 2005:

"I'm 17 and been feeling unwell since I was 15. My doctor told me I had M.E when I was 16, but this diagnosis has now been changed to Fibromyalgia. I am now feeling totally bewildered and unsure where to turn next.

Any advice would be greatly appreciated, but what I really need is some guidance on where to find resources and websites that provide easy to understand information on fibromyalgia, as my family have no idea what I am experiencing and I am finding difficult to explain. I am always tired, constantly feel like I have a migraine headache and unable to concentrate for long. I can't even wash myself properly without being in terrible pain and frequently I need help with this personal necessity. Things are just so bad, but I can't explain it.

I do try and stay positive and the doctor who recently diagnosed my FMS has been very helpful. I also have a lovely, sympathetic boyfriend and truly hope that things will improve, but I just don't know what happens now!"

Pippa (UK)

Reply:

Firstly, it is good news that you have now been correctly diagnosed has having fibromyalgia, and that you are trying to remain positive, and although this may be confusing at the moment, with more information you will learn to cope with your condition. Also by having the support of your boyfriend and family is a great help and by including them in your research so that they can learn to understand this condition is an important step to copying with FMS. I have emailed you some information, tips on how to explain your symptoms to your family and friends, and some resource links to get you started.

Email 2006:

"Hello,

While searching for answers online I came upon your site and wanted to say thank you for sharing your story. I am seeing a new doctor tomorrow morning in the hope that he can help. I received a massage, year ago and had a therapist tell me she believed I had fibromyalgia, but I ignored her comments and being a therapist myself I found many who came to me for treatment. The more I listened to their symptoms the more I realized it sounded as if they were telling me how I felt and not themselves! I again ignored the symptoms and continued taking the pain medication that another doctor was prescribing for headaches… although I now was taking them for much worse pain, all over the body.

I still ignored things, saying I was just lazy, overweight, needed to just stop whining and forget the pain and exhaustion… I cannot ignore it any longer and hope this doctor has answers. I guess all I would really like is for him to say 'YES' you do have FMS, and that I am not crazy or just plain lazy.

Well, thank you for your site and if you have any suggestions, please email me with them."

Peace Poet.

Reply:

Unfortunately, I have no answers. Just simply keep pushing your Doctor for a diagnosis and for some help. Then when you get a diagnosis try as many different treatments as you can to see if you can find one that helps. Think and be positive – as you and I understand the pain that you suffer. Those that do not have fibromyalgia or any other arthritic condition can not even start to understand how sufferers feel on a daily basis. You certainly are not lazy or crazy, just simply suffering from a condition that can not be easily recognized, diagnosed or treated. Finding people, including family and friends that are supportive is important in helping you cope through the worst days. I truly hope that your doctor will provide the answers you require, so that the correct treatment can begin and the pain management more effective.

Letter 2006:

"Dear AJ,

My daughter-in-law has suffered with fibromyalgia for 5 years now, since the birth of her second child. She has an addictive personality and so the drugs have become a big problem for her. Her addiction is preventing her from having the determination to learn how to cope and live with her FMS.

Your opening page of your website could have been written by her!

She is your age and feels much older, and doesn't have much hope and sees her future as a painful, abnormal life where she can not be the mum and wife she desperately wants and needs to be. She just got out of detox, for taking too many headache pills… She doesn't handle her anxieties very well (turns to the pills) right now.

I want to help her help herself. What helped you the most?"

Claudia (USA)

Reply:

Thankfully, your daughter-in-law has the support of you and your family, which is so important in helping her cope through the worst days. Her doctor needs to be pushed for more help, especially as she can easily become addictive to the medication she is on, and that all other possible illnesses are ruled out. Perhaps try a different approach as some alternative therapies and medications can be helpful and run less risk of them becoming addictive, unlike many conventional treatments. Coping with this condition is a daily battle, as is finding a treatment to help alleviate some of the symptoms.

Encourage her to set herself some daily targets to achieve, as this will help to keep her motivated. Start small and increase on them. It can be anything she wants to do.

I sincerely hope that you and your daughter-in-law find some answers which will help her to manage the pain more effectively, enabling her to enjoy her life and family, especially her children and husband.

"Little deeds of kindness, little words of love, help to make earth happy like the heaven up above."

Authors Final Word:

At this stage, I decided to write a brief update on my progress before sending this book off to be published.

In July 2006 I was sent to the Medical Physics Clinic in Grantham for a bone scan to see if any other causes could be identified that may be creating the excruciating pain that I suffer. This was quite a long day, with a 45 minute car journey one way, then the actual test being in two parts.

Part One: This half of the study took just 15 minutes and simply involved a small injection which contained a small amount of radiation in the form of a liquid. This meant that for safety, I had to avoid pregnant women and children for several hours throughout the day. Having had the injection, I was then required to wait for 3 hours before the second part of the test could be implemented.

Part Two: The second half of the study was the actual bone scan, where I was required to lie perfectly still during the scan so that a correct reading could be taken. The scan took 30 minutes and I must say that I was glad to get up and move around afterwards, as this was not the most comfortable procedure I have endured. Trying to be still when you are in pain is like trying to stop a leaf blowing in the wind… However, the results of the scan didn't reveal any abnormalities, but my Rheumatology consultant still wasn't happy with the way my joints are swollen and still believes that there may be a possibility of some form of arthritis, so he decided to send me to Lincoln hospital for an ultra-sound test of my small joints, etc, to see if this identifies any other conditions. If nothing was identified from this test, then my consultant had considered to continue to treat my symptoms as fibromyalgia and prescribe a new drug called Lyrica.

In the meantime my consultant changed my medication again as the new dosage of the drug co-codamol wasn't helping my symptoms it was just making me feel extremely nauseous. So he prescribed me with ***Buprenorphine Transdermal*** which, suppose to provide 24 hour pain relief in the form of a patch which is worn for 7 days before replacing with a new one. This new medication had very little effect at alleviating the pain, but that's nothing new! Most the medications I try have little effect, but we continue experimenting to see which ones do and don't help. This is why I am so keen to try alternative therapies alongside the conventional treatments, as most conventional drugs can't be that healthy and most have side effects attached to them anyway. So it's back to that old vicious circle again, cure one thing only to have it replaced with another.

Anyway, the most recent medications prescribed are as follows.
In September 2006 I was prescribed a combination of Tramadol Hydrochloride 50mg and Paracetamol 500mg, which tend to just numb some of the pain and discomfort for a short time until the dose starts wearing off. I can take up to 16 of these pain killing tablets daily.
At this point my consultant had completed all the tests possible and concluded that my condition may actually be osteoarthritis, but with the possibility of some rheumatoid arthritis which will be confirmed by a final set of blood tests and from the results of a steroid injection to see if the inflammation is reduced. Since November 2006 when the osteoarthritis was confirmed, but still inconclusive with regards to having rheumatoid arthritis, I was prescribed the drug Sulphasalazine 500mg (Salazopyrin ® En-Tabs)*, which are used to help reduce the symptoms and slow the progress of rheumatoid arthritis and other forms of arthritis by reducing the inflammation. It is still early stages to know whether this latest medication is having any affect as it can take up to 12 weeks for any benefit to be noticed, but I have to say I'm not too happy on some of the know side effects, such as the risk in the reduction of cells in the blood. 1 in 700 patients may suffer a serious fall in the number of white blood cells, of which the majority of such patients suffer from rheumatoid arthritis. My consultant is observing closely and blood tests during the first three months of treatment are recommended.

So from having years of fibromyalgia, I now have to cope with the symptoms of arthritis, but that is the high risk of having a family who suffer with various forms of arthritis and the inherent gene being passed through our family bloodlines to myself and other generations of our family.

My father always understood how I feel everyday and the pain that I suffer, as he too had osteoarthritis. On the 8th November 2006, a day before my 36th Birthday, I was given the terrible news that my dad had terminal cancer. The Melanoma (skin cancer via a mole on his leg) that he had removed earlier in the year had spread to my dads liver and lungs. Sadly, 3 weeks after being told the diagnosis my life, and that of my family was devastated on the 27th November 2006 when my dad died peacefully at home. Even though I was with him right to the end, I can't explain the pain and despair of losing not just my dad, but a friend who was always there for me. Thankfully I still have my mum, who also has arthritis and even through her own grief her support is never ending.

"Families are so precious, as is life. So cherish every moment."

Maybe one day a cure will be found for everyone suffering the pain of fibromyalgia and/or arthritis, but until then it is up to our selves and the medical profession to make life as comfortable as possible. It isn't easy and there will be times when you really do not feel like pushing yourself that little bit further. Maybe, that is how you feel today, but don't get disheartened, we all have days like that.

During the writing of this book, I had many days where I just hadn't got the energy or concentration to do more than a few lines, or it was too uncomfortable to sit in front of the computer and type. However, many months later this book has eventually been published and I am proud of my achievement and if it helps just one other person suffering from fibromyalgia or from the pain of arthritis, then I will be satisfied and very happy.

Just think positive, keep smiling and laughing and hopefully tomorrow will be a better day than today…

I asked God for a flower,
He gave me a garden.
I asked God for a tree,

118

> *He gave me a forest.*
> *I asked God for a river,*
> *He gave me an ocean.*
> *I asked God for a friend,*
> *He gave me You.*

Finally, I would also just like to thank all those in the medical profession who have offered help and support over the years, including:

Dr. Bryan – GP, Wombourne, Staffordshire (Appointments in 1999)

Dr. G. Kitas – Rheumatology Consultant, the Guest Hospital, Dudley, West Midlands (Appointments from 1999)

Dr. B. Stuart – Rheumatology Consultant, the Princess Royal Hospital, Haywards Heath, West Sussex (Appointments from 2001)

Dr. P. J. Dawson – GP, Swineshead, Lincolnshire (Appointments from 2006)

Dr. V. V. Kaushik – Rheumatology Consultant, Grantham & District Hospital, Lincolnshire (Appointments from 2006 – ongoing)

All the nurses and nuclear medicine technologists and to the physiotherapists that have all helped over the years. Your dedication and support is appreciated.

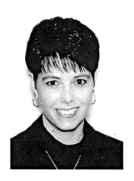

**God Bless &
Very Best Wishes
Angela J Coupar**

---

* Chapter Footnote: March 2007. I have been taking the Sulphasalazine for 4 months now and I'm happy to say that I have definitely seen an improvement in my condition. The pain is not as bad, with the exception of very cold or wet days. I am not as stiff and uncomfortable and even sleep better. The best thing is that I have been able to reduce my pain killers from 16 tablets per day to 8 tablets per day, which can only be a good progression. I truly hope that the Sulphasalazine continues to help and that my most recent blood tests have good results when I see my Rheumatology consultant at the end of April. For me, it doesn't matter if the medical professionals are unable to identify the exact form of arthritis that I have, as long as the medication continues to give me the quality of life that someone of my age expects…

Key Words

Analgesic: These are mediciations that relieve pain.

Arthritis: Simply meaning joint inflammation and is often used to indicate a group of rheumatic related conditions. Arthritis affects not only the joints, but also connective tissues such as the muscles, tendons and ligaments, and the protective layers of internal organs.

Auto-immune Disease: A condition where the immune system destroys, or attacks a persons own body tissue.

Cartilage: The tough, resilient tissue which covers and protects the ends of bones. Cartilage acts as our body's own natural shock absorbers.

Chronic Disease: Used to describe a pro-longed illness.

Collagen: This is the substance, or main structural protein of bone cartilage, connective tissues, skin and tendons.

Connective Tissue: The supporting structure of the body and its internal organs.

Fibromyalgia: A chronic condition that creates pain, discomfort and stiffness throughout the tissues that support and move the bones and joints. Pain and tender points are experienced in the muscles, particularly in the region of the neck, shoulders, spine and hips. A condition that creates widespread pain, fatigue and sleep disturbance.

Flare Up: The re-appearance or increase in symptoms.

Genetic Marker: A specific tissue type or gene, similar to a blood type that is transferred from parents to children. It is also known that some genetic markers are linked to conditions such as rheumatic diseases.

Inflammation: Heat, pain, redness and swelling associated to injury or disease.

Joint: A point where two bones meet. Joints are usually built up of cartilage, joint space, fibrous capsule and synovium.

Ligaments: These are a group of cordlike tissues that connect the bones to each other.

Muscles: These are groups of specialized cells that, when stimulated by the nerve pulses contract and produce movement.

Myopathies: The term used to describe inflammatory and non-inflammatory diseases of the muscles.

Non-steroid Anti-inflammatory Drugs (NSAIDs): These are a group of drugs used to reduce inflammation associated with joint pain, stiffness and swelling. *Example:* Aspirin.

Remission: The term used to describe a period during which symptoms related to disease are reduced (partial remission) or disappear (complete remission).

Sleep Disorder: The term used to describe the condition where a person has difficulty in achieving restful, restorative sleep. Combined with other symptoms, people suffering from fibromyalgia usually experience sleep disorders.

Synovium: This is a tissue which surrounds and protects the joints. It also produces synovial fluid which nourishes and lubricates the joints.

Tender Points: The term used to describe the specific areas on the body that are, painful especially when pressed.

Tendons: These are fibrous cords which connect muscle to the bone.

References

(1) Biochemist Harvey Kaufman sold his invention to the biochemist, Rik Deitsch who now licenses the product to an MLM company, selling it as a branded liquid health supplement. For more information on Zeolite visit the website: http://www.drzeolitedetox.com/natural-cellular-defense.html

(2) Dr. Gabriel Cousens, M.D., M.D. (H) Diplomate of the American Board of Holistic Medicine, Diplomate of Ayurveda & Director of the Tree of Life Rejuvenation Centre. The Natural Zeolite Product, Clinical Summary. http://www.liquidzeolite.org/gabriel-cousens.html

(3) Food Intolerance and nutritional information, and food intolerance tests available to purchase online from Dr. Gillian McKeith's website. http://www.drgillianmckeith.com

(4) AmsterdamKliniek provide downloadable (pdf) brochures on Allergies & Other Sensitivities, Fibromyalgia and Chronic Fatigue Syndrome (M.E.). http://www.amsterdamkliniek.com

(5) The Great Plains Laboratory in Lenexa, KS. Research information on the abnormally high levels of yeast and fungal metabolites in urine of fibromyalgia patients. (www.greatplainslaboratory.com/fibromyalgia.html)

(6) Wolfe F, Smythe HA, Yunus MB, Bennett RM, Bombardier C, Goldenberg DL, *et al.* The American College of Rheumatology 1990 criteria for the classification of Fibromyalgia. Report of the multi-centre criteria committee. Arthritis Rheum 1990;33:160-72

(7) Bennett RM. Fibromyalgia: Commonest cause of widespread pain
.   Compr Ther 1995;6:269-75

(8) Haugen M, Kjeldsen-Kragh J, Nordvag BY, Forre O. Diet and disease symptoms in rheumatic diseases – results of a questionnaire based survey. Clin Rheumatol 1991;10:401-7

(9) Hostmark AT, Lystad E, Vellar OD, Hovi K, Berg JE. Reduced plasma fibrinogen, serum peroxides, lipids and apolipoproteins after a 3-week vegetarian diet. Plant Foods Hum Nutr 1993;43:55-61

(10) K. Kaartinen, K. Lammi, M. Hypen, M. Nenonen, O. Hanninen, A. –L. Rauma. Vegan diet alleviates fibromyalgia symptoms. Scand J Rheumatol 2000;29:308-13

(11) C McGonigle, Surviving Your Spouse's Chronic Illness: A Compassionate Guide,(New York: Henry Holt, 1999).

(12) MJ Pellegrino, *The Fibromyalgia Supporter,*(Columbus, Ohio: Anadem Publishing, 1997)

(13) Pellegrino, The Fibromyalgia Supporter

(14) Arthritis Foundation, "Living and Loving: Information About Sexuality and Intimacy," (1993)

(15) L Barbach, *For Each Other: Sharing Sexual Intimacy,*(New York: New American Library, 1984)

(16) Arthritis Foundation, "Living and Loving," 2

(17) Pellegrino, Fibromyalgia Supporter, 65

(18) Pellegrino, Fibromyalgia Supporter, 66

(19) Herbal Remedies for Arthritis, Fibromyalgia, Muscular Aches and Joint Pains by AyurvedicCure.com. For more information and other herbal remedies visit the Natural Health website. http://www.naturalhealthweb.com/articles/AyurvedicCure2.html

(20) Fibrohugs Letter written by Ronald J. Waller – Copyright of Fibrohugs.com

(21) Study by professional lecturers and teachers, Dr Caroline Dott & Dr Andrew Dott on the effect of drugs and premature ejaculation. More information can be located at http://www.fmscommunity.org/nl40.htm

Recommended Fibromyalgia Related Publications

You may also find that these books and booklets are well worth reading. Most are available from leading bookshops and online bookstores.

Coping with Fibromyalgia (Fibrositis) - Written by Beth Ediger (Foreword by D L Goldberg, MD) - 38 pages (ISBN 0-9695785-0-4)

Fibromyalgia: Fighting Back - Written by Bev Spencer (Foreword by Dr. G McCain) - 40 pages (ISBN 0-9695785-2-0)

Both the above booklets are produced by LRH Publications, Toronto. To obtain these, try your local library, local support group, or an international book shop, such as Amazon on the internet. **They are also available from:** http://www.arc.org.uk

Fibromyalgia & Chronic Myofascial Pain Syndrome: A Survival Manual *(2nd Edition)* - Written By Devin Starlanyl, M.D. and Mary Ellen Copeland, M.S. M.A – New Harbinger Publications, 2001

Fibromyalgia: A comprehensive approach. What you can do about chronic pain and fatigue Written by Miryam Ehrlich Williamson - Walker & Co; New York, 1996

All About Fibromyalgia, A Guide for Patients and Their Families - Written by Daniel J. Wallace, M.D. and Janice Brock Wallace - Oxford University Press, 2002

The Womens Guide to Ending Pain, an 8-Step Program *(Info; on managing chronic pain including fibromyalgia)* - Written by Howard S. Smith, M.D. and Debra Fulghum Bruce - M.S. John Wiley & Sons, Inc; 2003

Fibromyalgia: Simple Relief Through Movement – Written By Stacie Bigelow – John Wiley & Sons Inc, 2000

The First Year of Fibromyalgia: An Essential Guide for the Newly Diagnosed (*The First Year Series*) **-** Written by Claudia Craig Marek - Marlowe & Company, 2003

Betrayal by the Brain: The Neurologic Basis of Chronic Fatigue Syndrome, Fibromyalgia Syndrome, and Related Neural Network Disorders - Written by Jay A. Goldstein – Haworth, 1996

Women Living with Fibromyalgia - Written by Mari Skelly - Hunter House, 2003

The Fibromyalgia Relief Book: 213 Ideas for Improving Your Quality of Life - Written By Miryam Ehrlich Williamson - Walker & Co; 1998

Effortless Pain Relief - Written by Dr Ingrid Bacci – Bantam, 2005

Fibromyalgia Syndrome: Fighting the Devil With the Patience of Job: (*A Victims Point of View & Survivors Guide*) - Written by Marilyn Sue - Xlibris Corporation, 2002

Fibromyalgia: Understanding and Getting Relief from Pain that will not Go Away - Written by Don L. Goldenberg, M.D. - Perigee, 2002

Recommended Arthritis Related Publications

Osteoarthritis: Your Questions Answered – Written By John Dickson & Gillian Hosie – Churchill Livingstone, 2003

Stop Osteoarthritis Now! Halting the Baby Boomers' Disease – Written By Harris H. McIlwain & Debra Fulghum Bruce – Simon & Schuster Ltd, 1996

All About Osteoarthrtis: The Definitive Resource for Arthritis Patients and their Families – Written By Nancy E. Lane & Daniel J. Wallace – Oxford University Press Inc, USA, 2002

The Expert Patient's Guide To Living A Full Life With Rheumatoid Arthritis –
Written By Jasmine Jenkins – How to Books Ltd, 2005

Rheumatoid Arthritis: The Infection Connection (Targeting and treating the cause of chronic illness) – Written By Katherine M. Poehlmann (Ph.D) – KF & KM Poehlmann, 2002

The Arthritis Bible: A Comprehensive Guide to Alternative Therapies & Conventional Treatments for Inflammatory Diseases – Written By Leonid Gordin – Inner Trade Bears & Company, 1999

The Doctors' Home Cure for Arthritis: The Best Selling, Proven Self Treatment Plan – Written By Giraud W. Campbell – Harper Collins, 2002

Treating Arthritis: The Drug Free Way – Written By Margaret Hills – Sheldon Press, 2006

Say No To Arthritis (Optimum Nutrition Handbook) – Written By Patrick Holford – Piatkus Books, 2000

Diet and Arthritis: A Comprehensive Guide to Controlling Arthritis

through Diet – Written By Gail Darlington & Linda Gamlin – Vermilion, 1998

Flax Oil as a True Aid against Arthritis, Heart Infarction, Cancer and other Diseases – Written By Johanna Budwig – Apple Publishing, 1996

The Arthritis Research Campaign publish, many free leaflets including:

Fibromyalgia
Introducing Arthritis
Osteoarthritis
Rheumatoid Arthritis
Blood Tests & X-Rays for Arthritis
Complementary Therapies
Hydrotherapy and Arthritis
Pain and Arthritis
Caring for a Person with Arthritis
Diet and Arthritis
Driving and Your Arthritis
Sexuality and Arthritis
Work and Arthritis, and
Your Home and Arthritis

They also provide information leaflets on the many drugs used to treat arthritis including:

Drugs and Arthritis (General Information)
Azathioprine
Cyclophosphamide
Gold by Intramuscular Injection
Local Steroid Injections
Methotrexate
Non-Steroidal Anti-Inflammatory Drugs
Penicillamine, and
Sulphasalazine

Fibromyalgia Resources:

The following resources contain information, advice and support associated to the condition Fibromyalgia that I have come across over the years and have found to be very helpful. However, I am not responsible for the content of these resources and can not make any representations regarding their content, or accuracy.

It's amazing the information you can find by simply searching the internet and exploring the benefits of search engines.

Fibromyalgia & Arthritis *(My own personal site, formerly Living with Fibromyalgia)* – http://www.fibromyalgiaandarthritis.co.uk

Association UK - http://fibromyalgia-associationuk.org

National Fibromyalgia Association (NFA) - http://fmaware.org/

Fibromyalgia Northern Ireland - http://www.fmsni.org.uk

Fibromyalgia Association UK - http://www.ukfibromyalgia.com

Website describing & showing fms tender points -http://www.fibromyalgia.com/tender_points.htm

Fibrohugs: *Support for sufferers and relatives, Information, Resources on Fibromyalgia and related illnesses such as MS & Lupus. National Fibromyalgia Spokesman is Larry Wilcox (Jon Baker) the actor from the TV series 'Chips'* - http://www.fibrohugs.com

FibroCare Center: *Information about Fibromyalgia and the Fibro Care Program offered at Point Chiropractic Center in Point Pleasant New Jersey, a balanced multifaceted program to help people who suffer from fms improve their quality of life* - http://fibrocarecenter.com

Fibromyalgia Financial Information - http://bcorsa.freeyellow.com/coping.html

Healing Well: *Information/Guides and Community sites on many diseases, disorders and chronic illnesses* - http://www.healingwell.com

Fibromyalgia Natural Products Centre - http://www.fmsyndrome.com/

Immune Support: *Several pages on fms including, Overview, Diagnosis,*
Treatment & Fibromyalgia Chat - **http://www.immunesupport.com/**

Fibromyalgia - http://www.0disease.com/0fibromyalgia.html

Fibromyalgia Syndrome (FMS) - http://www.lewolf.com/fms.htm

What in the world is Fibromyalgia? *(Several pages)* -http://www.plaidrabbit.com/fms/fibrom3.htm

Alternative & Conventional Treatments for Fibromyalgia *(several pages) -*
http://members.aol.com/_ht_a/fibroworld/alternative.htm

Fibromyalgia: A Guide for Patients - http://www.medhelp.org/lib/fm-pt.htm

Information site - http://www.fibromyalgia-symptoms.org/fibromyalgia_causes.html

Support for families of FMS sufferers - http://www.lclark.edu/%7esherrons/topic_consider.htm

A Guide for Family & Friends of FMS sufferers - http://www.sover.net/~devstar/relative.htm

Information Site - http://www.drpodell.org/fibromyalgia_treatments.shtml

FMS Site for Men - http://www.myfibrosite.com/users/dwaynebright/index.html

Men with Fibromyalgia – http://www.menwithfibro.com

Fibromyalgia Information Site - http://www.fibromyhelp.com/treatments.html

MSM (*Methyl-Sulfonyl-Methane*) - http://www.msm.com

Arthritis & Pain Relief Resources:

Arthritis Research Campaign (ARC) – http://www.arc.org.uk

Arthritis Care – http://www.arthritiscare.org

Arthritis Foundation – http://www.arthritis.org

National Rheumatoid Arthritis Society (NRAS) – http://www.rheumatoid.org.uk

Stiff UK – http://www.stiffuk.org

The British Pain Society – http://www.britishpainsociety.org.uk

The Pain Relief Foundation – http://www.painrelieffoundation.org.uk

Pain Concern – http://www.painconcern.org.uk

Other Helpful Links:

Say No To Cancer – Information on ZNatural *(The original patented product)* and how zeolite minerals may be beneficial to many health conditions and not just cancer, but arthritis, depression, etc. - http://www.saynotocancer.co.uk

Activated Zeolite Liquid – Information on Zeolites and its benefits – http://www.liquidzeolite.org/summary.html

Directory for Complementary Therapists in the UK & Northern Ireland –
http://www.uktherapists.com

Natural Health & Healing Directory, with practitioners & therapists representing 108 different countries – http://www.internationalholistic therapiesdirectories.com

Institute for Complementary Medicine – http://www.i-c-m.org.uk

Miscellaneous Links:

Canine Angels – http://www.canine-angels.co.uk

Hamster Rescue (UK), caring for old, unwanted and neglected hamsters, Information & Advice always available – http://www.hamsterrescue.org.uk

Authors Other Book:

Now Available at Amazon.co.uk & Amazon.com

Canine Behaviour Practice: A Short Guide to Setting Up your own business as a
Dog Psychologist, Behaviourist or Therapist.   By Angela J Coupar

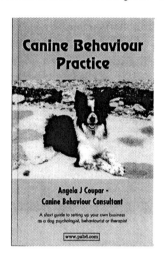

ISBN 1-905277-40-7

**Available as a
Paper Back Book
&
E-book (pdf format).**

Book Synopsis:

An easy to follow guide for anyone who is studying or recently qualified in the field of canine behaviour, or for those interested in finding out how to set up a canine behaviour practice.

Contents include: Considering a career as a canine behaviourist, health & hygiene, information on setting up and running a practice, behaviour advice, recommended reading and a helpful resource page.

For more information and to read the reviews on this book or too order directly from me, please visit my bookshop at:

http://www.canine-angels.co.uk

Original Paper Back copy – Priced = £9.99 including p&p (UK Only)

E-book (pdf format) – Priced = £4.99

Dedication:

A Final Farewell to my beautiful Canine Companions.

In Loving Memory of

William – Border Collie – Aged 18

1988 – 2006

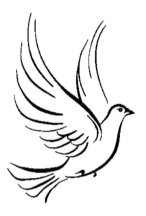

In Loving Memory of

Bracken – Border Collie – Aged 13 ¾

1990 – 2003

They helped me through the roughest days with a cuddle, a lick, a
paw to hold and listened for hours, just as true friends do.
Always Missed and Never Forgotten.

Printed in the United Kingdom
by Lightning Source UK Ltd.
121786UK00001B/178-189/A